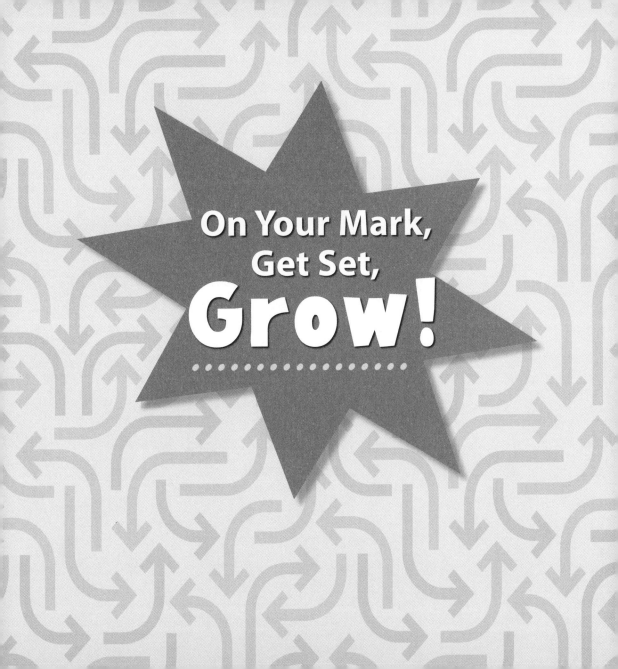

On Your Mark,
Get Set,
Grow!

Other Books in the "What's Happening to My Body?" Series

The "What's Happening to My Body?" Book for Boys

My Body, My Self for Boys

The "What's Happening to My Body?" Book for Girls

My Body, My Self for Girls

Ready, Set, Grow!
A "What's Happening to My Body?" Book for Younger Girls

My Feelings, My Self: A Growing-Up Guide for Girls

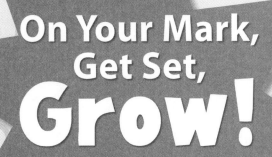

On Your Mark,
Get Set,
Grow!

A "What's Happening to My Body?"
Book for Younger Boys

Lynda Madaras

Illustrations by Paul Gilligan

Newmarket Press • New York

This book is published in the United States of America.

First Edition

10 9 8 7 6 5 4 3 2 1
ISBN: 978-1-55704-781-6 (pb)

10 9 8 7 6 5 4 3 2 1
ISBN: 978-1-55704-780-9 (hc)

Library of Congress Cataloging-in-Publication Data

Madaras, Lynda.
On your mark, get set, grow! : a "what's happening to my body?" book for younger boys /
Lynda Madaras ; illustrations by Paul Gilligan.
p. cm.
Includes bibliographical references and index.
ISBN 978-1-55704-781-6 (pbk. : alk. paper) — ISBN 978-1-55704-780-9 (hardcover : alk. paper)
1. Teenage boys—Growth—Juvenile literature. 2. Teenage boys—Physiology—Juvenile literature.
3. Puberty—Juvenile literature. I. Gilligan, Paul, ill. II. Title.
RJ143.M328 2008
613'.04232—dc22
2007043095

QUANTITY PURCHASES
Companies, professional groups, clubs, and other organizations may qualify for special terms when
ordering quantities of this title. For information or a catalog, write Special Sales Department,
Newmarket Press, 18 East 48th Street, New York, NY 10017;
call (212) 832-3575; fax (212) 832-3629; or e-mail info@newmarketpress.com.

www.newmarketpress.com

www.whatshappeningtomybodybooks.com

Designed by Jaye Medalia

Manufactured in the United States of America

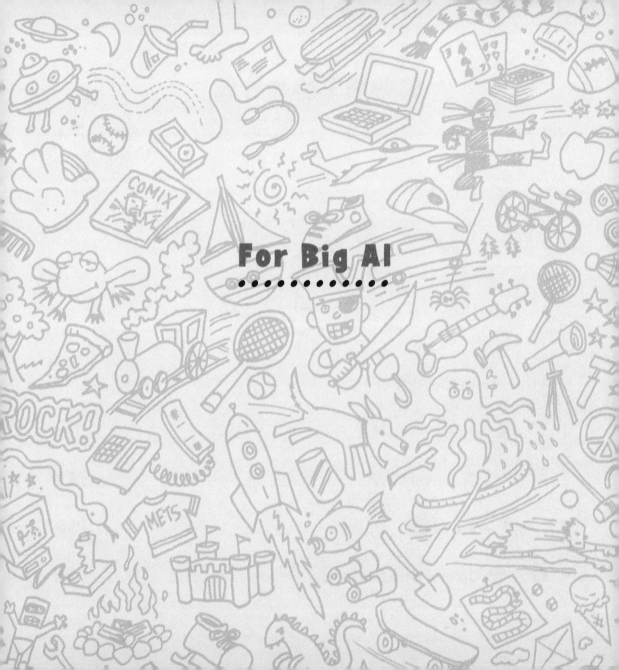

For Big Al

contents

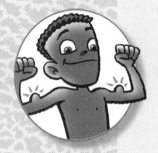
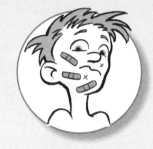
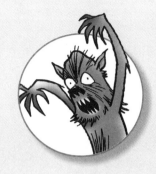

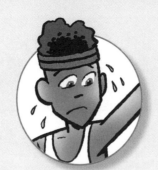

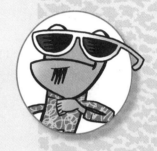

Note from the author

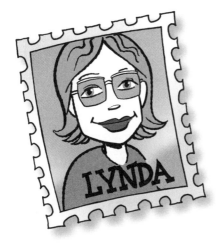

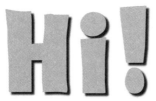

My name is Lynda Madaras.

· · · · · · · · · · · · · · · · · ·

I write books about growing up and going through puberty for boys and girls. I also teach puberty classes and workshops.

(Chances are, you already know what puberty is. But in case you don't, I'll give you a quick idea. Puberty is a time of changing. It lasts only a few years. But during this time your body changes from a child's body into a man's body.)

I wrote my first puberty book with my daughter, Area. (It's called The "What's Happening to My Body?" Book for Girls.) Area was going through puberty at the time. She helped me know puberty from a girl's point of view. My second puberty book was written for boys. Boys in my puberty classes helped a lot with that first boys' book. They helped me understand puberty from a boy's point of view.

Quite a few years have gone by since those first two books. Area grew up, went to college, and got a job. She fell in love. She got married, and now has two young daughters.

During these years, I've continued to write and teach about puberty. I've written more books about puberty. I've taught quite a few puberty classes. I've gotten thousands of letters from readers. My readers and kids in my

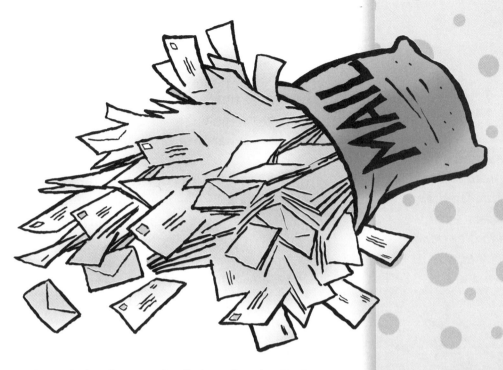

classes have helped me with all these books. In fact, many of the quotes in my books come from them.

When I was starting this book, I called up some of the boys who had been in my first puberty classes. Of course, they are grown up now. They had all gotten through puberty. But, as boys, they had helped me with my first boys' book. It was fun to get in touch with them. Some of them are now married and have sons of their own.

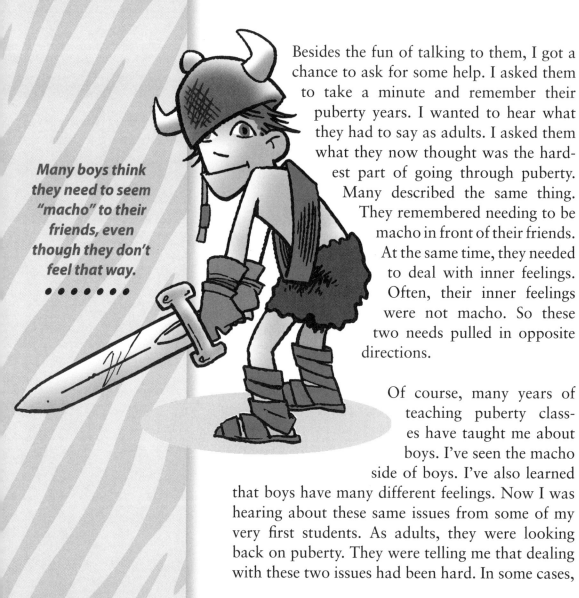

Many boys think they need to seem "macho" to their friends, even though they don't feel that way.

• • • • • • • •

Besides the fun of talking to them, I got a chance to ask for some help. I asked them to take a minute and remember their puberty years. I wanted to hear what they had to say as adults. I asked them what they now thought was the hardest part of going through puberty. Many described the same thing. They remembered needing to be macho in front of their friends. At the same time, they needed to deal with inner feelings. Often, their inner feelings were not macho. So these two needs pulled in opposite directions.

Of course, many years of teaching puberty classes have taught me about boys. I've seen the macho side of boys. I've also learned that boys have many different feelings. Now I was hearing about these same issues from some of my very first students. As adults, they were looking back on puberty. They were telling me that dealing with these two issues had been hard. In some cases, it was the hardest part of going through puberty.

Puberty has a way of bringing up strong feelings. You might be scared about changes that are happening to you. You might be confused about how you're supposed to act. You might feel the pressure of being pulled in two directions. You might be discovering romantic feelings.

Puberty may also increase the need to be macho. But it's pretty hard to live up to the macho, or "real man," image. According to this image, "real men" don't show their feelings. They are never confused, or uncertain, or afraid. But, of course, none of this is true. Real boys and real men do sometimes get confused. They do sometimes feel uncertain. They do sometimes feel afraid. And the truth is, hiding our feelings doesn't make them go away. In fact, it just makes them harder to deal with. That's why talking about feelings is important.

I hope this book will help you talk about puberty and your feelings about growing up. Maybe it will help you talk with your mom and dad. Maybe you can read it with them. Maybe you and a good

Puberty has a way of bringing up strong feelings.

friend can read the book together. As you read, you can talk about it.

I've been writing puberty books and teaching classes for more years than I want to say. During this time I've talked to a lot of boys. Most boys don't hold back. They tell me just what they're thinking and feeling. They ask questions about what happens during puberty. They also tell me how they feel. Many of the things they say are here in this book. Many of their questions are here, too, along with my answers. So, in a sense, boys like you helped write this book. So have boys like you who are now grown up.

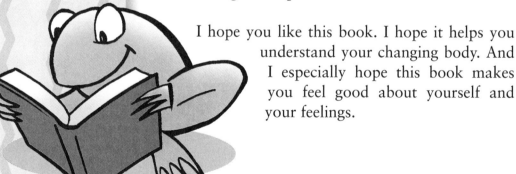

I hope you like this book. I hope it helps you understand your changing body. And I especially hope this book makes you feel good about yourself and your feelings.

What's Happening to Me?

Puberty Is About Change

● ● ● ● ● ● ● ● ● ● ● ● ● ● ● ● ● ●

You're growing up. Of course, that's nothing new.
After all, you've been growing up all your life. Ever
since the day you were born, you've been growing
in many ways. Year by year, you've been growing
bigger. You've been getting taller and heavier. But
this growing up is different.

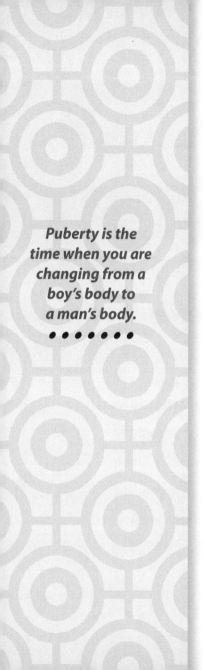

Maybe you've noticed that your sex organs are getting larger. Maybe you're seeing some hairs in places that were bare before. Hair may be growing around your sex organs. This hair is called pubic hair. Or maybe you're getting erections (hard-ons) more often.

> The **scrotum** (SKROW-tum) is a loose bag of skin that hangs behind the penis.

Has any of this stuff happened to you?
If so, you may be asking, "Am I weird?"

No! You are not weird. You are 100% NORMAL! You're just starting puberty.

What if none of this has happened to you yet? Does that mean you're weird?

No! You are not weird, either. You are 100% NOR-MAL, too! You haven't started puberty yet, but you will. Sooner or later all of us start puberty.

What Is Puberty?

Puberty is a special time in a boy's life. During puberty, a boy's body changes into a man's body.

This doesn't happen all at once. Puberty takes time. From start to finish, puberty may take anywhere from two to five (or more) years.

How does puberty start? What happens first?

In boys, puberty starts when their **testicles** and **scrotum** begin to develop. The testicles and scrotum grow larger and hang lower. Testicles, or balls, are two egg-shaped organs. They lie inside the scrotum. The scrotum is the sack of skin behind the penis. Not all boys notice these first changes. For them, pubic hairs are the first sign of puberty.

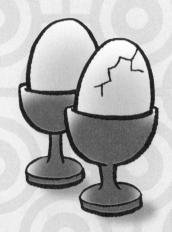

These changes are just the start. Many others follow. Maybe you already know about these changes. In my puberty classes, we make lists of these changes. I divide the class into teams. Each team has an outline of the male body. They also have a bunch of markers.

"On your mark, get set, go!" I say, and each team writes as many changes as they can. Then I say, "Stop." The team with the longest list wins. On the next page is one winning team's list.

You may not know what some of these words

List of Changes
●●●●●●●●●●●

Pubic hair

Growing really fast

Bigger muscles

Shoulders wider

Hair under your arms

Darker hair on arms
  and legs

Penis grows

Testicles develop

Mustache

Beard

Start shaving

Sweat more

Voice changes

Body odor changes

Zits, pimples, acne

More erections

Begin to ejaculate

Wet dreams

mean. Not to worry! This book will teach you about all these changes.

As you can see, puberty is a time of many changes. The kids in my classes have lots of questions about these changes. Chances are, you do, too. That's what this book is all about—answering your questions about growing up.

When Does Puberty Start?

Boys don't all start puberty at the same age. Some

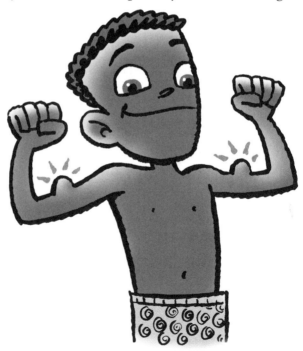

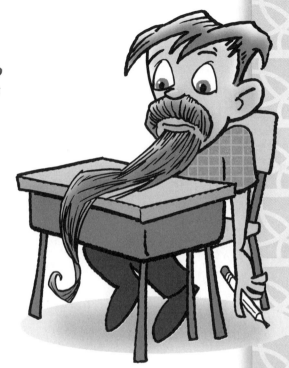

No matter how it may seem, your body is growing up at the speed that's right for you. We each develop according to our own timetable.

• • • • • • • •

boys start when they're only eight. Some start even earlier. Others don't start until they're almost fifteen.

❝ Being late paid off in the end. I'm fifty and I still look young. Some of my friends had beards in the eighth grade. Now they're hammered. ❞

❝ You know, I thought I was late. But now I see that it wasn't true. Really I was about average, or maybe even early. ❞

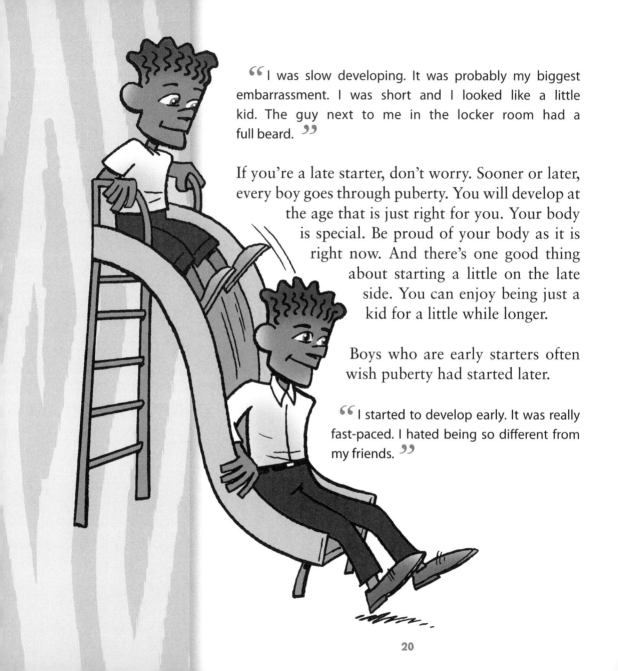

> **"** I was slow developing. It was probably my biggest embarrassment. I was short and I looked like a little kid. The guy next to me in the locker room had a full beard. **"**

If you're a late starter, don't worry. Sooner or later, every boy goes through puberty. You will develop at the age that is just right for you. Your body is special. Be proud of your body as it is right now. And there's one good thing about starting a little on the late side. You can enjoy being just a kid for a little while longer.

Boys who are early starters often wish puberty had started later.

> **"** I started to develop early. It was really fast-paced. I hated being so different from my friends. **"**

Your body is growing up at the speed that's right for you. In a few years, you and your friends will all have started puberty. Then it won't matter who was first or last. After all, we all end up in the same place—grown up!

Feelings About Puberty and Growing Up

66 It wasn't something that all of a sudden happened one day. Puberty kind of snuck up on me. It just happened bit by bit. 99

66 I got my first pubic hair in the fourth grade. I was pumped. 99

66 Puberty is kind of scary. Sometimes I think about it all and I go, 'Whoa! Slow it down.' 99

66 I was getting my first pubic hair. My brother started kidding me. So I always covered up when I came out of the shower. I felt shy. 99

You may feel really proud about starting puberty. Or you may feel shy. You may be a little scared

Growing Up Doesn't Mean You're a Grown-Up

• • • • • • • • •

When puberty starts, you might think that now you have to act differently.

"Everybody says, 'Puberty means you're becoming a man.' But I just want to go on being a kid. You know, goofing off and stuff like that. I'm not ready to be an adult."

You may feel this way, too. But puberty doesn't happen all at once. True, you are growing up. But (see next column →)

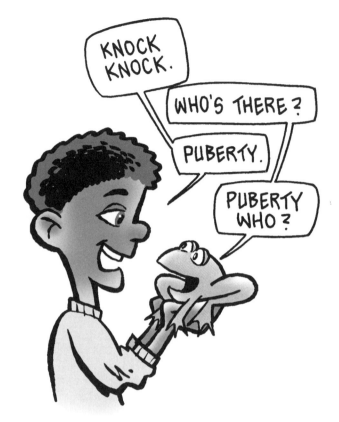

thinking about all the changes. You may feel one way one time, and another way another time. Feelings are like that.

When you're feeling proud, enjoy that feeling. Hold your head high. If you have some scared or shy feelings, take heart. You're not alone! Other boys are feeling the same way. We all go through the same changes. We all make it!

For most of us, puberty is a mixed bag. Sometimes you'll feel great. Other times, you may not feel so great. That's part of growing up.

Fact is, puberty isn't always a piece of cake. But there are things you can do to make it a little easier. Be prepared. Read this book. Better yet, read it with your mom or dad. Or read it with an adult you trust. Ask questions. Get the facts. Know what's happening to your body. Puberty is a lot easier when you know what to expect.

You can also read this book with your friends. Talk about puberty changes. Tell jokes. Talk about how you feel. The more you know and talk about it, the easier it will be!

that doesn't mean you have to be a grown-up. You've got lots of time yet. Your body may be changing. But you can still be a kid. You can still climb a tree. You can still be "just friends" with girls. You can act goofy. You can still play kid games.

You can be grown up for a time. Then you can act like a kid again. You can watch cartoons one day and MTV the next. You can do whatever you feel like doing. It's up to you. Be what you want to be.

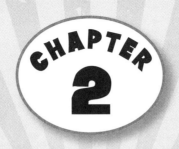

CHAPTER 2

Growing Up Down There
Your Sex Organs Are Growing

• • • • • • • • • • • • • •

66 My brothers told me what would happen. Then it did. My balls started getting bigger! Finally!! 99

66 I wasn't all excited or very happy about developing. I guess I just wasn't ready. I felt really out of it. 99

66 I wasn't really aware of my sex organs growing. It wasn't until I got pubic hair. Then I started paying attention. Then I saw that my balls were bigger. 99

Maybe you will notice when your sex organs first start growing. Or maybe you won't. Maybe you'll be happy about it. Or maybe you won't be so happy. Either way, sooner or later, your sex organs will begin to grow.

Your Sex Organs

The sex organs on the outside of your body are the **penis** and **scrotum**. Your **penis** has a shaft and a wider tip called the **glans**. Your scrotum is a bag of skin. It hangs behind your penis. Inside the scrotum are two egg-shaped organs. These are your testicles.

Boys have lots of slang names for the penis. "Dick" is one of these. There are slang names for the glans, too. It's sometimes called the "head." Also, there are lots of slang names for the testicles. "Balls" and "nuts" are just two. You can probably think of lots more.

> The **penis** (PEE-nis) has a shaft and an enlarged tip called the **glans** (GLANZ).

> *" The first change I saw was my balls hanging lower. And they weren't so tight. Everything was just looser and lower. I thought, 'This is puberty. This is great.' "*

Growth of Your Sex Organs

Your sex organs grow larger during puberty. This growth starts with your testicles and scrotum. This is the beginning of puberty for boys. Later your penis will grow larger.

The growth of your sex organs doesn't happen overnight. For most boys it takes two to five years. But some boys take less time. And some boys take longer.

Doctors talk about five stages of sex organ growth. Look at the pictures on pages 28 and 29. Can you tell what stage you are in? (These pictures show a boy who hasn't been circumcised.)

Circumcision (sir-kum-SISH-un) is an operation that removes the **foreskin** (FOUR-skin).

Circumcision

The pictures of the five stages show boys who have not been circumcised. **Circumcision** is an operation that removes the **foreskin**. The foreskin covers the glans. It is a special part of skin of the penis.

The operation is usually done when a baby is only a few days old. Sometimes it is done for religious reasons. In the past, most male babies in this country were circumcised. Now, only about six out of ten babies are circumcised. It's different in other countries. There, babies are usually circumcised only for religious reasons.

In grown men, the foreskin can be pulled back over the glans. This is true for some boys, too. But other boys can't pull it back all the way. If you can't, don't worry. Over time it will loosen up. Then you will be able to pull it back. But don't ever force the foreskin back!

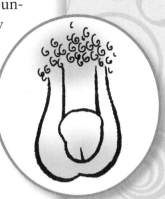

circumcised

Keep It Clean

Maybe you have a foreskin, or maybe you don't. In any case, you need to wash your sex organs every day. Use a mild soap and water. If you have a foreskin, gently pull it back and wash the glans and the whole foreskin. If soap stings, it's OK to use just plain water. If you can't pull your foreskin back, don't worry. Just wash the outside of the foreskin.

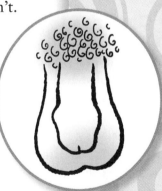

uncircumcised

More about penis size in Chapter 7.

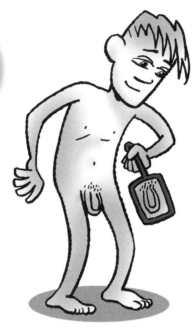

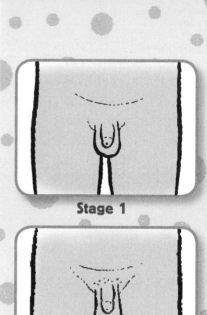

Stage 1

Stage 2

Stage 1 **Childhood**

This is the stage before puberty begins. Your sex organs do not change very much during childhood. Your body grows. But your sex organs grow only a little. They don't grow very much until puberty starts.

Stage 2 **Puberty Starts**

Stage 2 starts when the testicles and scrotum begin to enlarge. The biggest change is in the size of these sex organs. The penis itself doesn't get much larger. The scrotum gets longer. It also reddens or gets darker. The testicles hang lower. The skin of the scrotum gets thinner and looser. It is more baggy and wrinkled.

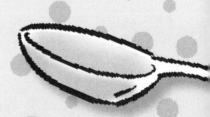

This spoon holds about 4 ml.

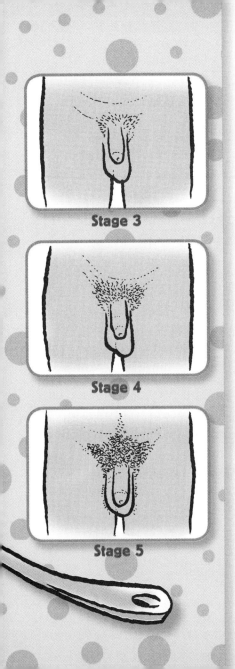

Stage 3

Stage 4

Stage 5

Doctors can measure the size of the testicles. If a boy's testicles are 4 ml (short for milliliters) or larger, he has probably reached Stage 2. This may happen anytime between his eighth and fifteenth birthdays. Some boys begin to grow pubic hair during Stage 2. Others don't start until later.

Stage 3 The Penis Grows Longer

The penis grows longer during Stage 3. But it doesn't get much wider. The testicles also grow more during this stage. The skin of the penis gets darker. The scrotum grows and continues to darken. Many boys start to grow pubic hair in Stage 3.

Stage 4 The Penis Grows Wider

The penis grows wider during Stage 4. Also, the glans develops. The penis continues to grow longer. But the major changes are in its width and in the glans. The skin of the sex organs continues to darken. The testicles keep growing. The scrotum hangs lower.

Most boys already have pubic hair when they start Stage 4. But some don't grow pubic hair until they are in Stage 4.

Stage 5 Adult

The testicles are fully grown. They are usually between 14 and 27 ml in size. The scrotum is also fully developed. The penis is now fully grown.

Questions & Answers

Q Both of my testicles started growing at the same time. But now the left one hangs a lot lower. Is this normal?

A Yes, this is normal. For most boys the left testicle hangs lower. And the right one is a little larger. Sometimes it's the other way around. Either way is perfectly normal.

Q What should I do if I get hit in the testicles and the pain is really bad?

A Right after it happens, apply cold. Cold compresses or an ice bag are good. It's also good to lie down. If the pain starts to let up in an hour or so, that's good. There is probably no serious damage. But call your doctor or go to the emergency room right away if the pain gets worse. Do the same if any of these things happen:

- The pain doesn't let up in an hour.
- There's bruising or swelling.
- It's difficult to pee.
- You have bloody pee.
- Your pee is pink.

But prevention is best. Playing sports makes getting hit in the testicles more likely. So you should wear a jockstrap or other type of athletic protection. Ask your coach what kind is best for you.

Q **I have a brown circle around my penis. It's always been there. What is this?**

A I'm guessing you are circumcised. If so, I'd say this is the scar from when your foreskin was removed.

Q **I have only one testicle in my scrotum. It's been this way all my life. Should I see a doctor?**

A Yes. Talk to your mom or dad and see a doctor. You may be worried about seeing a doctor. Don't be. Your doctor won't be embarrassed at all. It's a doctor's job to help you take care of your body. And that means all parts of your body.

Q **I think I'm in Stage 3. Now something weird is happening with my voice. Sometimes it gets all high and squeaky. Is this part of puberty?**

A Yes, it is. During puberty your vocal cords grow thicker and longer. This makes your voice get deeper. While the vocal cords are growing, your voice may sound high-pitched and squeaky at times.

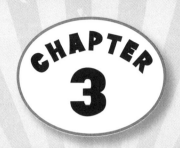

CHAPTER 3

Hair, There and Everywhere

All About Body and Facial Hair

• • • • • • • • • • • • • • •

Puberty is a hairy time! You sprout new hairs here and there. Places that were bare before suddenly have hair. All at once, you're a hairier you!

Now don't get me wrong. I'm not saying you will turn into Werewolf Boy overnight. But during puberty you do grow new hair on certain parts of your body. This chapter will tell you where and when to expect this new hair.

Pubic Hair

66 I saw pubic hair on my older brothers. They had more hair than me. And I said, 'When is it going to come to me?' 99

66 All my friends had pubic hair. But I didn't. It was embarrassing. I even thought about using my mother's hairnet. You know, gluing it in place above my penis. I even practiced looking at it in the mirror. It didn't look too bad. But then I thought about what would happen if the guys caught me with a pasted-on hairnet. That was the end of my plan to use my mother's hairnet. 99

66 Ugh, I didn't want it to get all hairy. I didn't want to get pubic hair. 99

Pubic Hair Stages

The first few pubic hairs are just the start. You grow more as puberty continues. As with genitals, there are five stages of pubic hair growth. Can you tell which stage you're in?

Stage 1 Childhood

You may have fine, short hairs growing on the belly and other places. But these are *not* pubic hairs.

Stage 2 First Pubic Hairs

The first pubic hairs begin to grow. There aren't very many of them. Most boys get their first pubic hairs when they're eight and a half to fifteen. But it can happen earlier or later than this.

Stage 3 Still Growing

The pubic hairs are curly and darker. There are more of them. They cover a wider area.

Stage 4 More Curly and Wiry

There is more pubic hair than in Stage 3. The hairs are dark, curlier, and wiry. They form a triangle. But they don't cover as wide an area as they will in Stage 5.

Stage 5 Adult

The pubic hair forms a bushy triangle. It reaches to the edge of the thighs. In some men, it grows out onto the thighs. It may also grow up toward the belly button.

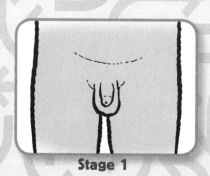

Stage 1

Stage 2

Pubic hair is often the first sign of puberty that a boy notices.

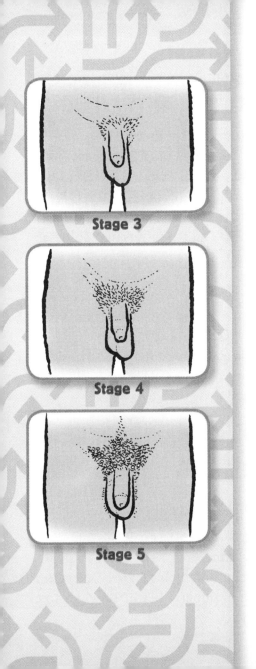

Stage 3

Stage 4

Stage 5

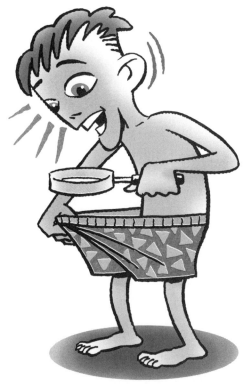

Your stage of pubic hair growth may not be the same as your stage of sex organ growth. The two things don't always go hand in hand. You could be in Sex Organ Stage 3, but only in Pubic Hair Stage 2. Or you might be in Pubic Hair Stage 4, but only in Sex Organ Stage 2. Don't worry if these stages don't match up. It's perfectly normal!

You may be glad to get pubic hair. Or you may not. But everybody grows pubic hair. It is all part of growing up.

Grown men have a triangle of short, curly hair growing around their sex organs. It's called pubic hair. Some men have a lot of pubic hair. Others don't have so much. Pubic hair may be red, black, brown, or blond. It may not be the same color as the hair on your head. When you are old, it may turn gray.

During puberty, boys begin to grow their first pubic hairs. These first hairs are more straight than curly. They may not have much color. There aren't many of them. You may have to look very closely to see them.

Pubic hair starts to grow sometime after the sex organs start to develop. It is often the first sign of puberty that a boy notices.

Underarm and Body Hair

During puberty, hair also starts to grow in your armpits. For most boys, underarm hair starts to grow a year or two after the first pubic hairs. But some boys are near the end of puberty before they get any underarm hair. And some get underarm hair first.

The hair on your arms and legs changes during puberty, too. Before puberty, this hair is soft and fine. It doesn't have much color. During puberty, it gets thicker. It also gets darker. There may be more of it.

Darker hair may also start to grow on your chest. Some boys grow hair on their shoulders, backs, or buttocks. Some grow hair on the backs of their hands. Some are really hairy. Others have very little body hair. Just how much hair you'll grow depends on your family background.

Facial Hair

"I had a very light beard at about 14. I started to shave then. But it was only once every three or four days. **"**

Your sex organs will likely be well developed before you see your first whiskers. Often they appear during Stage 4 of sex organ development. For most boys it happens between the ages of thirteen and sixteen.

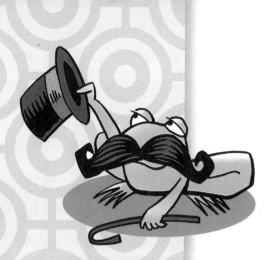

Usually, your first facial hairs will appear at the outer corners of the upper lip. At first, there won't be many. And they may not be very dark in color.

As a boy matures, his facial hair will get thicker and darker. His beard and mustache may be the same color as the hair on his head. Or they may be a different color. By age eighteen, your beard may be as full and

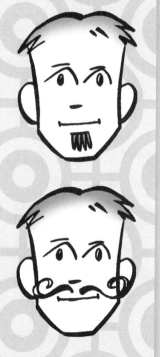

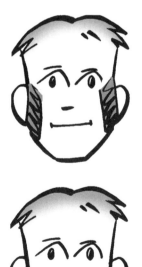

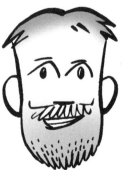

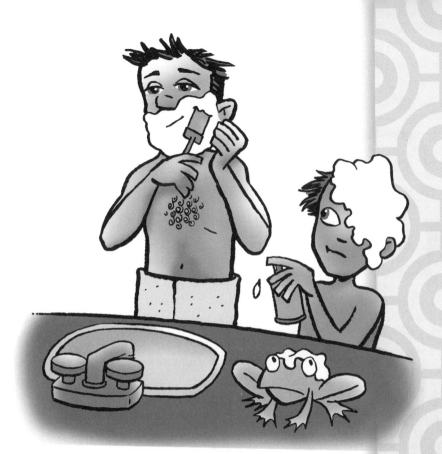

thick as it's ever going to be. But many men keep developing more facial hair into their twenties.

Some Tips on Shaving

❝ I like to watch my dad shave. He's really fast. ❞

❝ My older brother helped show me how to shave. It was cool. ❞

As you mature, your facial hair will get thicker and darker.

• • • • • • •

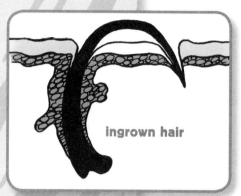

ingrown hair

Shaving with a blade razor cuts hair at an angle. It leaves hairs with sharp tips. These tips can curl back into the skin. This can cause painful bumps. To avoid this problem, always shave in the direction the hair grows.

"I used my father's razor the first time I shaved. I got in trouble for that. His razor was all messed up when he went to use it. I was excited when I first started shaving. But now shaving is a drag. So I let my beard grow."

There are different kinds of razors. Some men use an electric razor. Others use a razor with a blade. Most guys start out with plastic throwaway razors. They're easy to use. You just throw the whole razor away when the blade gets dull. But throwaway razors get dull after only a few shaves. So you may switch to a razor with a replaceable blade. With these, you replace only the blade and its holder or just the blade itself.

Be careful when you first shave. You don't want it to turn into a bloody mess.

It's easy to cut yourself while shaving. Also, blades can scrape the skin and cause "razor burn." This is a painful, red rash. A dull blade can pull on the skin, causing razor burn. Get some advice. This can come from your dad, older brother, or a friend.

Use warm water to wet the hair first. Then use a shaving cream or gel. Give the water and shaving cream a few minutes to work. This softens the hair and cuts down on razor drag. Don't use plain soap. It dulls the blade. And you won't get as smooth a shave. You want the blade to slide smoothly over your skin.

Shaving in the direction the hair grows is easier on the skin. On most of your face, you can shave downward, with the hair growth. But some men shave upward under their chins. This gives a smoother shave, but is harder on the skin. Never shave against the hair growth if you are prone to ingrown hairs.

African-American men may have problems with razor bumps. They may have tight, curly hair. African Americans' skin is also more likely to form scars, called keloids. If you're subject to keloids, be very careful. Even a little nick from shaving could leave a noticeable scar.

Here are a few more tips to help you shave safely:

● Go slowly and go easy. Don't mash or grind the razor into your skin. Don't go over the same spot again and again. It's no sin if you don't get every last hair.

● Make sure your blade is clean, sharp, and free of nicks. Dropping a razor can cause nicks you can't see. If you drop it, change to a new blade.

● Blades may get dull after four to five shaves. Change them often.

● Rinse the hair from your blade often while you're shaving. And rinse your razor well when you're done.

● After shaving, rinse the area with cool water. Then pat (don't rub) your skin dry. Your skin is very sensitive after shaving.

● Never lend or borrow a razor. This can spread germs.

Questions & Answers

Q I've just started to get pubic hair and I'm only nine years old. My friends kid me about it. Am I OK?

A Yes! You are OK. Lots of boys your age have pubic hair. There's not much you can do about your friends kidding you. You might as well just laugh along with them. After all, your friends are going to get pubic hair, too. And then you'll all be in the same boat.

Q I don't have much hair on my body. I don't have much pubic hair or chest hair. I'm Asian. Do you think that's why?

A It's likely that you will grow more pubic hair before you are an adult. But we are not all the same. Some men do have more pubic hair than others. The amount depends partly on race and ethnic background. Some Asian men do have less pubic hair than men from other groups.

Q I found some pubic hair in my underwear. Is it normal for pubic hair to fall out?

A Yes. Hair on all parts of the body is always being lost. Then new hairs grow to replace them. The same is true of your pubic hair.

Q **Does shaving make your mustache grow in faster?**

A No. But it may look as though it does. Your hair has thin tips and is thicker toward the bottom. When you first shave, you cut off the thin, hard-to-see tips of your hair. As the hair grows back, you don't see the thin tips. You just see the thicker part of your hair.

Q **I have a few hairs on my upper lip. I only shave every couple of weeks or so. Is there any way to make facial hair grow faster?**

A There's no way to make your facial hair grow faster. But you're young. Many boys don't reach full facial hair growth until their early twenties. You're perfectly normal. It's just that you will have to wait a while longer.

Q **My pubic hair is straight. There's a lot of it, so I know I'm past Stage 2. Shouldn't it be curly?**

A Most people's pubic hair is curly. But everyone is different. Your pubic hair may get curly as you continue to grow. Or it may stay straight. Either way, it's perfectly normal.

Q **I see all these different kinds of razors. Which is best?**

A There are many different kinds of razors. Some are electric; others are throwaway, cartridge, and razors with single, double, triple, and even quadruple blades. You should talk to your dad or your brother or a friend about what is best.

CHAPTER 4

Growing Up and Up and Up!

The Height Spurt

• • • • • • • • • • • • • •

Puberty is a time when we grow up...and up...and up! Of course, we grow taller all during childhood. But we grow much faster during puberty. This time of really fast growth is called the height spurt.

More about growing bones and body building in Chapter 5.

"I was 5 foot 2 and about 110 pounds. I was the shortest one in my class. Then suddenly I grew a whole foot. And in just 18 months I was 6 foot 2. I was the tallest in my class.**"**

Most boys don't grow a foot in a year and a half. But they all go through a height spurt during puberty.

The Height Spurt

Most children grow about two inches a year. Once the height spurt begins, growth speeds up. A boy may grow four inches a year. That's twice as fast. Some boys grow even faster!

The height spurt lasts a few years. Then growth slows back down. Most boys add nine to eleven inches during their height spurts. But we aren't all the same. You may grow more or less than this.

During the height spurt, the ends of your leg and arm bones are growing. The ends of these bones are soft. Serious injuries could occur at the soft ends of these bones. So you have to be careful, especially with bodybuilding exercises.

When a boy has finished growing taller, the soft ends of the long bones will harden. For most boys, this happens between the ages of sixteen and eighteen. When this happens, a boy is no longer prone to injuries at the growing bone ends.

Feet First

During the height spurt, all your bones grow. But some bones start their growth spurt before others. Guess which bones start first?

You guessed it! It's the bones in your feet. Your feet can be almost full-grown early in the height spurt.

66 My feet are growing so fast. I get new shoes. I hardly even get them broken in. They're too small. I need new ones. My mom says she's gonna go broke buying shoes. 99

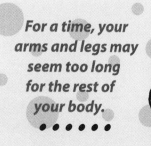

For a time, your arms and legs may seem too long for the rest of your body.

• • • • • • •

When their feet grow quickly, some boys worry. They think they'll end up with a closet full of Nikes. But there's no need to worry. Your feet won't keep on growing so quickly. They will slow down while the rest of your body keeps growing. Soon your body catches up with your feet.

Long Bones Next

Feet grow first. Then the long bones grow. Long bones are the bones in your arms and legs. They start to grow before the main part of your body. So your arms and legs may seem too long for the rest of your body. You may feel clumsy or klutzy. If so, don't worry. The rest of your body will soon catch up. And your arms and legs will be just the right length.

Girls First

❝You know when you're young and you're in fifth grade? You're 5 feet 2 and all the girls are 5 feet 7 or 8. You feel like a shrimp.❞

Girls go through a height spurt, too. Most girls start their height spurts around the age of 10. Most boys don't start before the age of 12 or 13. That's why 11- and 12-year-old girls are often taller than boys their age. Then boys start their growth spurt. Most of them soon catch up to and pass the girls. Look around at adults. Aren't most men taller than most women?

Most boys catch up to and even grow taller than girls. But it's also important to remember that tallness, or shortness, runs in families. So if your mom and dad are tall, you're more likely to be tall. And if your mom and

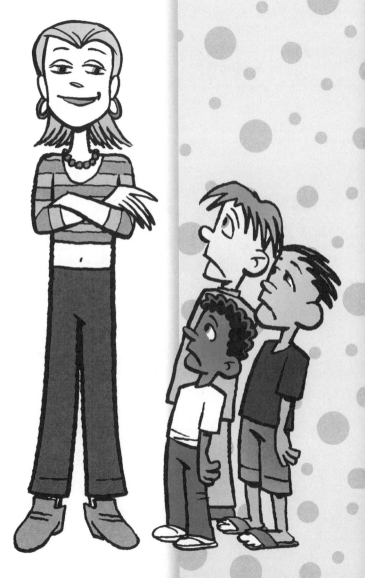

You can't do much about your height.
• • • • • •

dad are kind of short, you may be short, too. But, of course, that's not always true.

Too Tall? Too Short?

Some boys are unhappy about their height. They feel they are "too tall" or "too short."

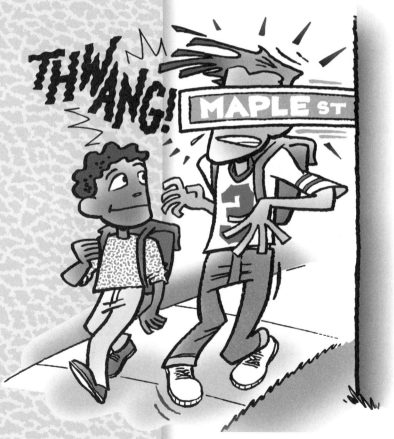

THWANG!

MAPLE ST

Being different from the other kids isn't always easy.

❝ I'm really tall. I think I'll go out for basketball. Sometimes people make jokes about my height. Then I wish I wasn't so tall. But mostly, I just dream of playing for the Lakers. ❞

Boys who are on the short side often wish they were taller.

" I'm short. I hate it. I always have to look up to people to talk to them. I'd give anything to be taller. **"**

If you're short, remember that you may not have completed your height spurt. You may still have quite a few inches to grow. Still, some boys do grow up to be shorter than they'd like. Fact is, you can't really do much about your height. What matters is the way you deal with it. You don't have to be tall to be a good friend. You don't have to be tall to be funny or smart or popular. You can't change your height. But you can go out there and be all the things you want to be.

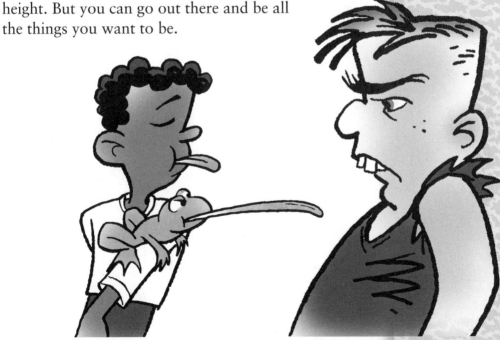

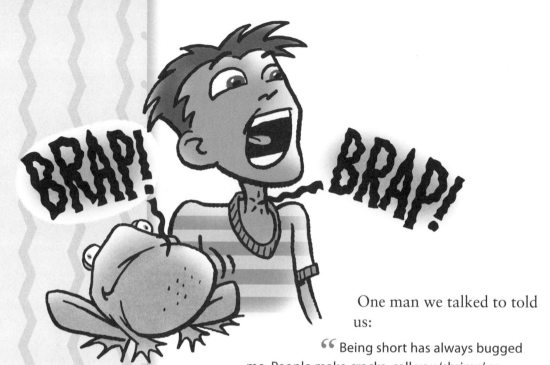

For more on "Voice Changes," see page 31 in Q&A.

One man we talked to told us:

66 Being short has always bugged me. People make cracks, call you 'shrimp' or 'shortie.' I'm really good at sports. Being short made it difficult to get on the team. I compensated by getting into weight lifting and wrestling. I still work out. I'm in great physical shape. A lot of guys my age are out of shape. I'm healthier than a lot of guys. Maybe if I'd been taller, I wouldn't have gotten into working out and taking care of my body. 99

How Tall Will I Be?

No one can tell for sure how tall you'll be. But there are a couple of clues.

Here's one clue. Has your height spurt begun? If you're tall before the height spurt, then you're likely to be a tall man. If you are short as a child, it's likely you'll be a short man. But it doesn't always work this way. Some boys are short before puberty. Then the spurt kicks in. They end up being among the tallest boys in their class!

Here's another clue. Is your dad no more than 5 inches taller than your mom? If so, you will probably grow to be at least as tall as your dad.

Did one clue say you would be tall? Did the other say you'd be short? Well, we never said they were perfect! They are only clues, after all.

Growing Strong Bones

During the height spurt, your bones grow quickly. Your grow-

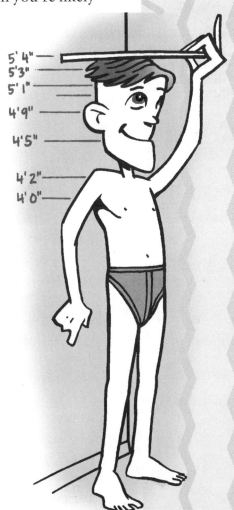

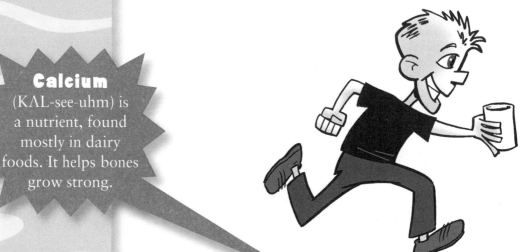

Calcium (KAL-see-uhm) is a nutrient, found mostly in dairy foods. It helps bones grow strong.

ing bones need lots of **calcium**. Calcium makes bones strong. Not getting enough can stunt your growth. It can weaken your bones. As we get older, our bones get weaker. You must get enough calcium while you're young. There's no way to make up for missed calcium later on in your life. Many boys your age are only getting about half the calcium they need.

Make sure you get plenty of calcium now. How? Get lots of calcium in your diet and plenty of exercise. Drink low-fat milk instead of soda pop. Eat foods that are rich in calcium. Cheese and yogurt are good choices. Calcium is now added to some

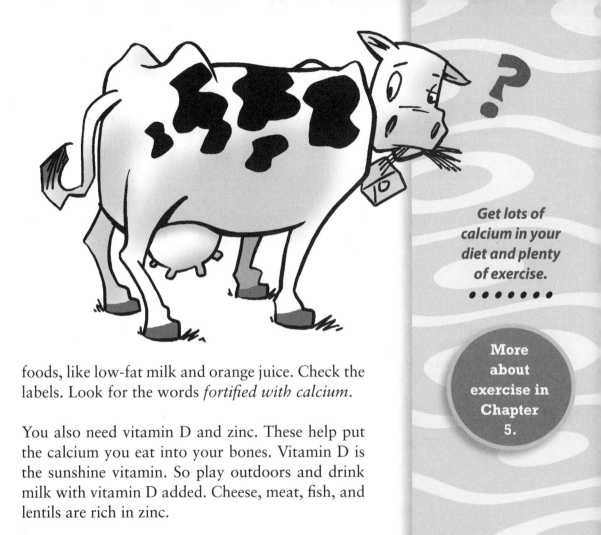

Get lots of calcium in your diet and plenty of exercise.

More about exercise in Chapter 5.

foods, like low-fat milk and orange juice. Check the labels. Look for the words *fortified with calcium*.

You also need vitamin D and zinc. These help put the calcium you eat into your bones. Vitamin D is the sunshine vitamin. So play outdoors and drink milk with vitamin D added. Cheese, meat, fish, and lentils are rich in zinc.

You need exercise, too. It helps the calcium you eat get into your bones. So don't be a couch potato. Get up. Shake a leg and get going.

Questions & Answers

Q **I get these pains in my arms and legs. They say they're just growing pains. What are growing pains?**

A Growing pains are a dull, achy kind of pain. Doctors don't really know what causes them. They happen most often around the age of thirteen. But younger or older boys can have them, too. They can happen in the arms or legs, or other parts of the body. Growing pains come and go. Sooner or later, they go away and don't come back. If the pain is always in the same place, see a doctor. Or if it's not a come-and-go kind of pain or if it's really bad, see a doctor.

Q **What is scoliosis?**

A Scoliosis (skoh-lee-OH-sis) is not a common problem for boys. But it does happen. When it happens the spine curves in an abnormal way. In most cases you just need regular check-ups to make sure it doesn't get worse. Sometimes you have to wear a brace for a while. It's easiest to deal with the problem when it's found early. So if your hips and shoulders aren't level or your spine curves, check it out with a doctor.

Q I'm the shortest boy in my class. Is there anything I can do to make myself taller?

A There's nothing you can do to make yourself taller. But give yourself time. Chances are, you still have some growing ahead of you. Try not to worry too much. Even if you don't get much taller, that's OK, too.

Q Does drinking coffee or smoking stunt your growth?

A Drinking coffee or tea will not stop you from growing. But you do need calcium for your bones. Don't let coffee or tea take the place of low-fat milk or other calcium-rich drinks.

Smoking won't stop you from growing. But smoking is worse for you during puberty. Your body is working hard to grow so fast. It is less able to cope with the poisons from smoking.

Q I'm really short for my age. People make cracks about how short I am. What should I say?

A It is hard to deal with rude people. It doesn't matter what they are being rude about. You could be polite and answer the rude question. You could ignore it. You could say, "I don't answer rude questions." You could tell them off. People may not mean to be rude. They just don't think before they open their mouths. You might let them know their question isn't nice. There are some people who are rude on purpose. They just have bad manners. They really are not worth worrying about.

Looking More Like a Man
The Weight and Strength Spurts

• • • • • • • • • • • • • • • •

You get taller faster during puberty. You also have an extra-fast gain in your weight. Part of this weight spurt is due to the growth of your bones and organs. Part comes from the bigger muscles you grow. Your shoulders get wider. This makes your hips look narrower. All in all, you look more like an adult man.

The Weight Spurt

The weight spurt is like the height spurt. It is a time of extra-fast growth during puberty. It happens at about the same time as the height spurt.

The weight spurt lasts a few years. A boy may gain 20 pounds in just one year. In all, most boys add about 45 to 50 pounds. Of course, we're not all the same. You may gain more or less than this. Some kids think they're getting fat. It's really just the weight spurt kicking in.

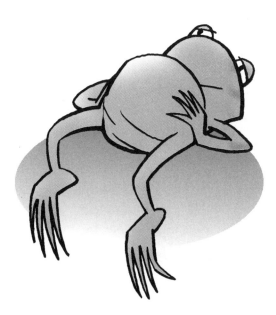

The Strength Spurt

A boy's strength increases during puberty. During this time boys become stronger than girls. Their muscles grow bigger.

Pound for pound, your muscles become stronger than a girl's muscles. During puberty, your muscles change in a special, male way. This change makes them work better. And it makes them even stronger.

Your muscles won't get stronger right away. First your muscles get bigger. Then, a few months later, they start getting stronger. This change in muscle strength usually comes later in puberty. It comes after the height and weight spurts. It continues into the early twenties.

During puberty, your muscles change in a special, male way. They work better and they get stronger.

• • • • • • •

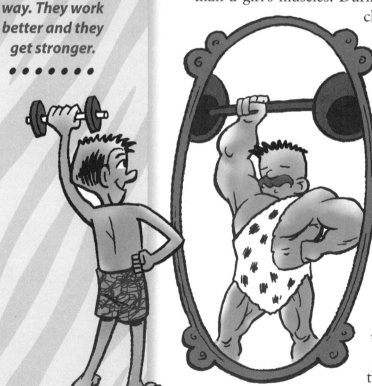

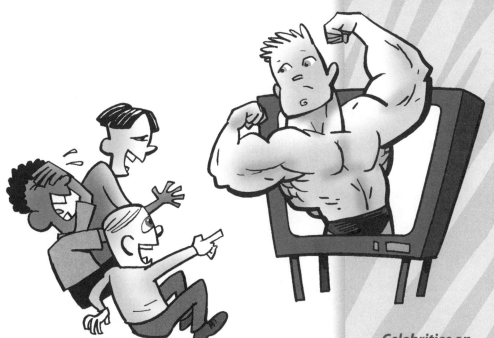

Bodybuilding

" I like the way I look, but I'm not really muscular. My friends all want to be totally buff. "

It's great to have big muscles. It's great to be in good shape. But there are other reasons boys want to be buff. We all see lots of actors on TV and in the movies. Many have really muscular builds. They have muscular chests and arms and legs. We see them on billboards and in magazines. We see them over and over and over again. They send a message.

Celebrities on TV and in the movies may make you think that a super-muscular body is normal for a man.

• • • • •

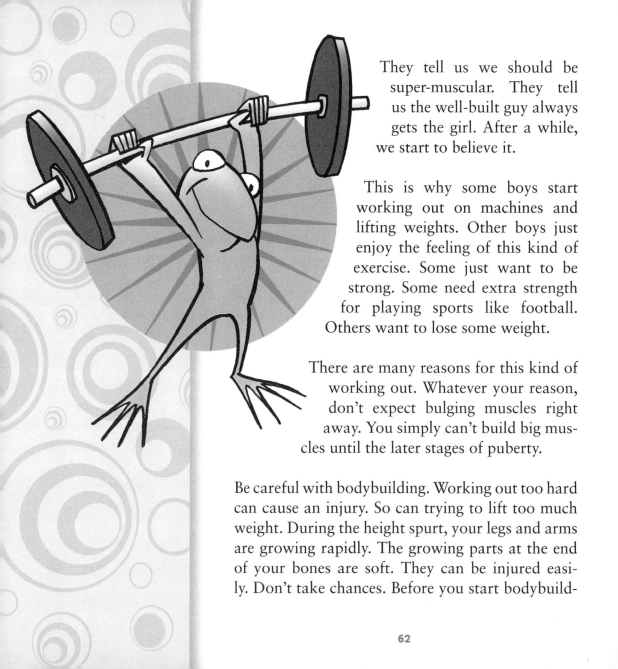

They tell us we should be super-muscular. They tell us the well-built guy always gets the girl. After a while, we start to believe it.

This is why some boys start working out on machines and lifting weights. Other boys just enjoy the feeling of this kind of exercise. Some just want to be strong. Some need extra strength for playing sports like football. Others want to lose some weight.

There are many reasons for this kind of working out. Whatever your reason, don't expect bulging muscles right away. You simply can't build big muscles until the later stages of puberty.

Be careful with bodybuilding. Working out too hard can cause an injury. So can trying to lift too much weight. During the height spurt, your legs and arms are growing rapidly. The growing parts at the end of your bones are soft. They can be injured easily. Don't take chances. Before you start bodybuild-

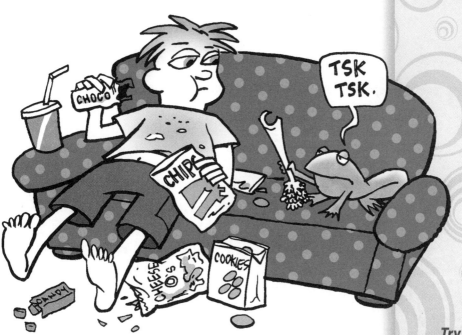

ing, talk with a doctor. Your doc can tell you what's right at your stage of puberty. Work with a coach or trainer on a safe program. Stay within the guidelines they set.

Eating Smart

Give your body the energy it needs to grow. Eat enough to satisfy your hunger. Don't eat too much of any one thing. Eat a variety of foods at meals

Try not to eat too much junk food. It's high in sugar, salt, and fat and low in nutrients.

• • • • • • •

and snacks. That way, you'll be sure your body gets everything it needs. That's eating smart!

Try not to eat too much junk food. Junk food has a lot of sugar or fat (or both!). It doesn't have the nutrients you need. You can't grow strong and healthy on a diet of chips, cookies, candy, and french fries. So make smart food choices. After school, don't wolf down that bag of chips or cookies. Snack on celery sticks with peanut butter. Or have an apple or a bowl of berries. Find something healthy you really like to snack on.

Here are some more tips to help you eat smart and be fit.

Think About Drinks

Cut down on sodas and sugary fruit drinks. Drink LOTS of water. How much water you need depends on how big you are. But try to drink between four and eight glasses of water every day. Fat-free or low-fat milk is a good choice, too. Milk has protein and calcium. You need that calcium for strong bones. (Remember we talked about calcium in Chapter 4.)

Snack on Fruits and Veggies

Snack on fruits and raw veggies. Apples, bananas, strawberries, and melons are great. Try vegetables raw. Grate carrots or beets to top off a sandwich or salad. And don't forget the leafy green veggies, like spinach and lettuce.

Eat More Grains

Cereal, bread, rice, and pasta are all grains. They give you energy. They also have fiber and vitamins.

Kids who eat a good breakfast are more alert.

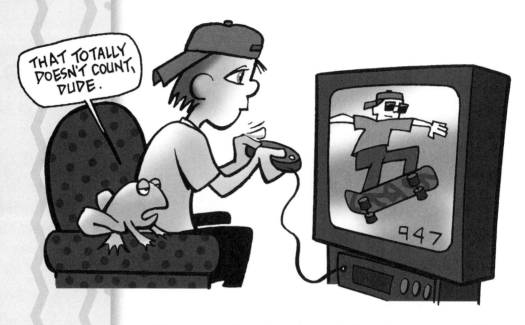

Eat smart by choosing whole wheat over white bread. Skip the sugary cereals. Choose oatmeal and other sugar-free cereals.

Don't Skip Breakfast

You need energy to stay alert and learn in class. It's a fact. Kids who eat a good breakfast do better in school. They are more alert. They are also less likely to be fat. So start your day with a good breakfast. Try fruit with yogurt or cereal and low-fat milk. Whole-wheat toast and whole-grain waffles are smart choices.

Cool It on Junk Food

You can still munch on junk once in a while. No one's perfect. Cookies and chips are OK from time to time. But you need to eat smart most of the time. Say you have a candy bar or cookies at lunch. That's fine. But try to even things out. Choose a fruit or veggie for your after-school snack. Get used to eating lots of good foods. After a while, you may not feel like eating the junk foods as much!

And Exercise, Too

Eating smart is one key to a healthy body. Exercise is another. We all need exercise. It helps you be your best weight. It burns up the food you eat so it doesn't get stored as fat. But it does more than just keep you thin. It makes your heart and lungs stronger. It also helps put calcium in your bones. So get off the couch and start moving around!

As we get older, most of us slow down. Adults are less active than teens. Most adults and teens just don't get enough exercise. Teens are less active than young children. It's normal to slow down as you grow older. But most people slow down too much. Guess when this slowdown happens? You're right. The slow-

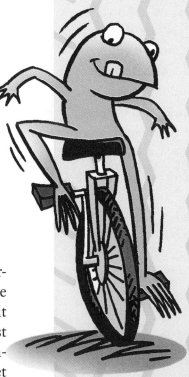

Don't stop riding your bike. Keep climbing trees and running around like a little kid. Stay active.

●●●●●●●

down often comes during the puberty years.

Don't let puberty turn you into a couch potato! Don't stop riding your bike. Keep climbing trees and running around like a little kid. Stay active. Get the exercise you need. Join a sports team at school. Run around the track. Make it fun. Start a hiking club. Learn to ride a unicycle.

How much exercise should you get? You should be active every day. That might mean games, sports, walking, or dancing. Anything that keeps you moving.

You should get 60 minutes of exercise on most, or better all, days of the week. Do something that really gets you moving. You need to breathe hard. You need to get the heart pumping fast. Try fast walking, running, or biking. Join a team, like track and field or baseball or football. Sports like swimming and tennis are also great. You don't have to be super jock. But you do have to make the effort.

Get in the habit of being active.

Questions & Answers

Q How much of the different food groups should I eat each day?

A There's not one answer for everybody. It depends on your age and your level of activity. To find out what's right for you, visit www.mypyramid.gov/kids. Find the list of subjects on the left side of the screen. Then go to "My Pyramid Plan." On the next screen, enter your age, sex, and physical activity. Then hit "submit." The next screen tells you how much of each food group you should eat.

Q My best friend is muscular and looks great at the beach. Girls just come up to him and start talking. But me, I'm just tall and skinny. I've been through my height and weight spurts. But I just don't have big muscles.
How come?

A I don't know exactly what stage of puberty you're in. You may have some more muscles to grow. But facts are facts. Some boys are born to be muscular. And some aren't. Oh sure, you can work out and build up some muscles. And that's great! But there are three basic body shapes. Some boys are tall and thin. Some boys tend to be on the stocky side. And some boys are muscular and athletic. We can't change our basic body shape. So if you're tall and skinny, don't plan to play center on the football team. Work with what you've got. Lots of girls like tall, thin guys. Trust me.

Q **I like to work out. At the gym some of the older guys talk about steroids. I don't think they're using steroids. But they're talking about how steroids build bigger muscle. But they're bad for you, right?**

A You bet they're bad. Some steroids are made by the body. And they are OK. But the steroids used by some bodybuilders are man-made. And they are bad news, especially during puberty. Here are just some of the ways they can hurt your body. They can stunt your growth. They can shrink your testicles. They can make your breasts grow larger. They can cause moodiness. They can cause "roid rage." This is a term used by bodybuilders. It means sudden and strong outbreaks of anger.

Q **I'm in puberty. I'm supposed to be looking more like a man. But I'm really freaked out. My breasts are getting bigger. Am I turning into a girl?**

A No, you are not going to change into a girl. Most people think that breast changes only happen to girls. They're wrong. Boys' breasts don't change as much as girls' do. But they do change. The nipple gets larger. The ring of colored skin around it gets wider. Many boys also have some swelling of one or both breasts. It may last as long as a year or two. This swelling is normal. It happens to about half of all boys going through puberty.

CHAPTER 6

B.O. and Zits

A Survival Guide

• • • • • • • • • • • • • • • •

I can see where puberty is part of growing up. But do you have to have pimples and B.O. and greasy hair?

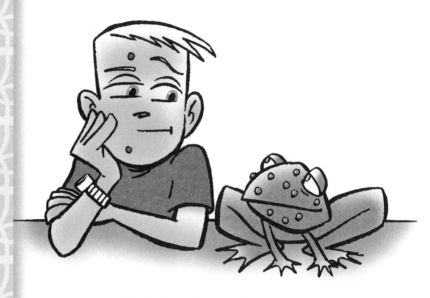

B.O. and zits can be part of growing up. But you can do something about them.

• • • • • • • • •

B.O. (smelly body odor) and zits (pimples) are NOT FUN! They're not on anyone's list of Great-Things-About-Growing-Up.

But during puberty you do sweat more. You also start to make a new kind of sweat. This new sweat changes your body odor. Your skin also makes more oil. This often leads to pimples.

No boy wants pimples or, worse yet, B.O. Still, they can be a part of growing up. But don't worry! This chapter will fill you in on how to treat pimples and avoid B.O.

Sweat and Body Odor

Sweat is natural and healthy. It helps keep you cool when you get too hot. Sweat, by itself, has no odor. But sweat does play a part in   body odor.

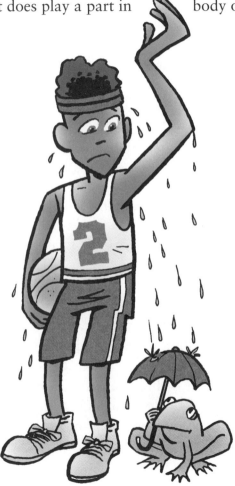

Here's a Tip
· · · · · · · · · ·

Wear 100% cotton clothes. Cotton "breathes." In other words, it lets air in. Your body stays drier under cotton clothes. There's less chance for B.O. germs to do their stinky work.

73

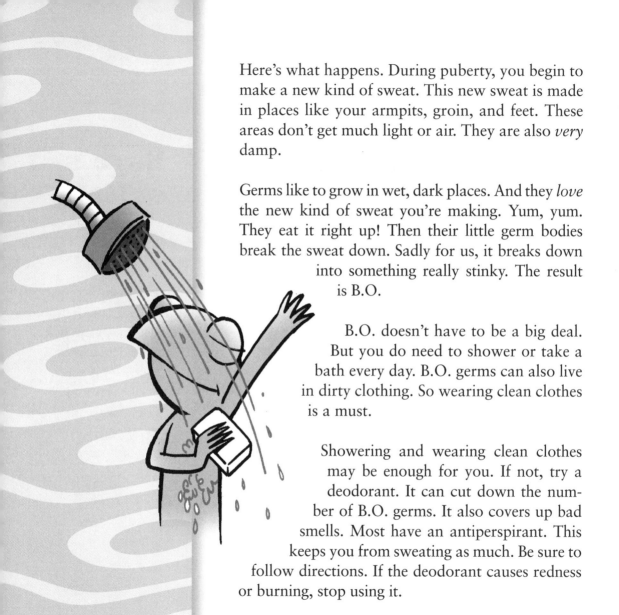

Here's what happens. During puberty, you begin to make a new kind of sweat. This new sweat is made in places like your armpits, groin, and feet. These areas don't get much light or air. They are also *very* damp.

Germs like to grow in wet, dark places. And they *love* the new kind of sweat you're making. Yum, yum. They eat it right up! Then their little germ bodies break the sweat down. Sadly for us, it breaks down into something really stinky. The result is B.O.

B.O. doesn't have to be a big deal. But you do need to shower or take a bath every day. B.O. germs can also live in dirty clothing. So wearing clean clothes is a must.

Showering and wearing clean clothes may be enough for you. If not, try a deodorant. It can cut down the number of B.O. germs. It also covers up bad smells. Most have an antiperspirant. This keeps you from sweating as much. Be sure to follow directions. If the deodorant causes redness or burning, stop using it.

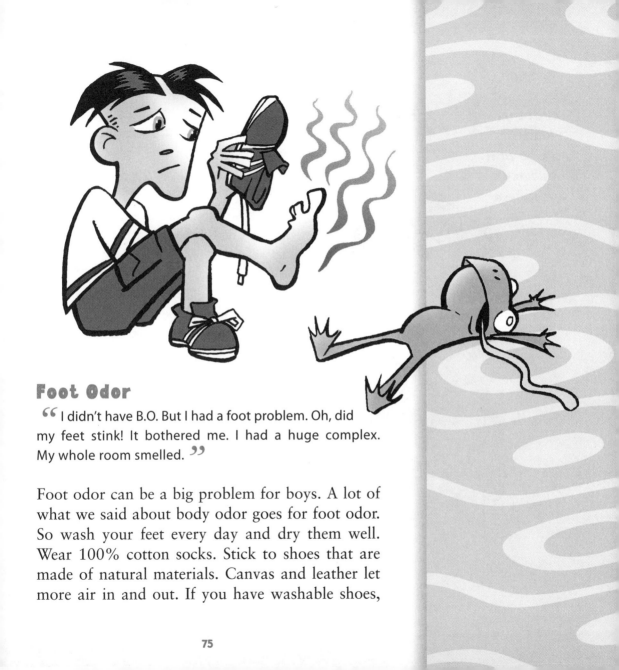

Foot Odor

" I didn't have B.O. But I had a foot problem. Oh, did my feet stink! It bothered me. I had a huge complex. My whole room smelled. "

Foot odor can be a big problem for boys. A lot of what we said about body odor goes for foot odor. So wash your feet every day and dry them well. Wear 100% cotton socks. Stick to shoes that are made of natural materials. Canvas and leather let more air in and out. If you have washable shoes,

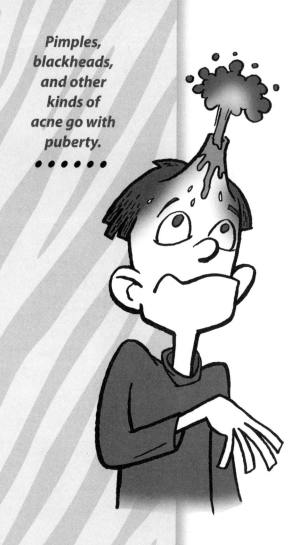

Pimples, blackheads, and other kinds of acne go with puberty.
• • • • • •

throw them in the laundry. Give your shoes a rest. Don't wear them two days in a row. Powders or sprays for the feet may help. You can also try deodorant shoe inserts.

Pimples

"I have the once-in-a-while whopper pimple. I have blackheads. But I don't have really bad acne."

"I've got really gross acne, really gross. I wash my face all the time. It doesn't help. I watch what I eat. That doesn't help, either."

Pizza, fried foods, and chocolate don't cause pimples. Washing your face a lot won't help. Pimples, blackheads, and other kinds of acne go with puberty. Here's why.

You have lots of oil glands. They're in almost every part of your skin. During puberty these glands make more oil. You also have little openings in the skin, called *pores*. They allow oil from the glands to get out onto the skin. The oil helps keep your skin soft. The oil also carries away dead cells from inside the pores. During puberty you make extra amounts of oil. You also shed more dead cells inside the pores. Dead cells and oil plug up the pores. Oil gets trapped. This trapped oil causes pimples, whiteheads, blackheads, or bad acne.

Even though the pore is plugged up, the gland keeps making oil. Pressure from the oil pushes the plug out of the pore. Bingo! You've got a whitehead. Blackheads look like tiny bits of dirt under the skin. They're not. They are trapped oil that has turned black. Germs can grow in trapped oil. This causes an infection that results in red, swollen pimples. The infection may spread under the skin. There may be large, red, painful bumps on your skin.

Now for the good news. There are things you can do about these skin problems.

Dealing with Pimples and Acne

Don't pop (squeeze) your pimples. You may spread germs and make your skin worse. Also, popping may leave scars that don't go away.

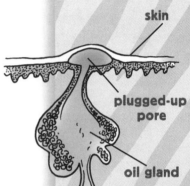

skin

plugged-up pore

oil gland

Your skin is making more oil. It's important to keep your skin clean. But twice a day is enough. Wash your face in the morning and again at bedtime. Don't scrub. Be gentle. Use a mild soap. Pat (don't rub) your face dry.

If you play sports or get real sweaty during the day, you could wash again. But don't overdo it. Washing more isn't going to clear up your acne. Washing can't get at oil trapped *under* your skin. And it's this trapped oil that causes pimples. In fact, too much washing can make things worse. Your skin may get too dry. Then the glands in your skin start making more oil. The result may be even more pimples.

Benzoyl peroxide (BEN-zoyl puh-ROK-side): A lotion you can buy in a drugstore that helps clear up acne.

At the drugstore, you can buy lots of products for pimples. Read the labels. Look for the words **benzoyl peroxide**. It's the best acne treatment you can get without a doctor's prescription. It fights germs and unblocks pores. It takes some time before you see results. In most cases, it takes about two weeks. But it may take as long as two months. If you don't see results by the end of two months, see your doctor.

Follow the directions. Don't just treat the pimples

you have now. Also treat the places where you've had problems in the past. Don't stop treatment when your skin clears up. If you do, the pimples may come back.

Be careful. Benzoyl peroxide can cause itching and redness. It may even make your skin worse at first. It comes in three strengths—2.5, 5, and 10 percent (2.5 percent is the mildest; 10 percent is the strongest). Start with the mildest. It will be less likely to bother your skin. After a while, your body may adjust to the medicine. Then, if you need to, switch to the 5 percent strength. Later, you may need the 10 percent strength.

Questions & Answers

Q My hair is greasy all the time. Is this because of puberty?

A Yes, it *is* because of puberty. There are glands in your skin that make oil. At puberty, they start to work overtime. They make more oil than ever before. Oil glands in your scalp start working harder, too. They make your hair oilier. You need to shampoo more often than you did before.

Q I don't know. Is my acne bad enough to see a doctor?

A Ask yourself these questions. Have you used a drugstore treatment for two months or more, but it hasn't worked? Do your pimples keep you from enjoying your life? Do bad cases of acne run in your family? Did your acne start when you were only nine or ten? Do you have large, red, painful bumps that don't go away? Does your acne leave scars?

Did you answer "yes" to any of these questions? If so, you should see a doctor about your acne.

Q My acne is bad. It's really a bummer. My parents just say, "Oh, you'll grow out of it." What can I do?

A True, most of us do grow out of it. But what about the time between now and then? Besides, you don't want to risk ending up with scars. You may want to see a doctor.

Talk to your parents about seeing a doctor. Take your time. Try to explain to them how much it means to you. You might try writing a letter. It's often easier to make your case in writing. You might also want to show them the answer to the previous question.

Q Is it normal to have zits other places than on my face?

A Yes. Pimples can occur anyplace where there are oil glands. They often show up on the neck, back, chest, and shoulders. These pimples are the same as the pimples on your face. You can treat them in the same way.

Q My friend has B.O. Should I tell him?

A If you don't, someone else will. And that person might not do it as kindly as you will. How you go about telling him is important. It will have a lot to do with how he takes it. It's best done in private, not in front of a group.

Q My sister and I have a bet. I say boys get more pimples than girls.

A You win.

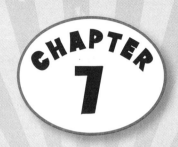

CHAPTER 7

What's Up Down There?

All About Erections

• • • • • • • • • • • • • • • •

Your penis is stiff and hard. It stands out from your body. Your scrotum gets tighter. Your testicles pull up closer to your body. What's happening? You're having an erection! "Boner" is a slang name for an erection. When it's erect, the penis is very stiff and hard. It can seem as if there's a bone in there. But there's not.

"Boner" is just one of the slang names for an **erection.** There are lots of others. Hard-on, woody, and stiffy are just a few. You can probably think of more. But, no matter what you call them, you'll have them more often during puberty.

Males have erections all their lives. Even tiny babies get erections. But during puberty they happen much more often. Let's take a look at how an erection happens.

Erections: The Inside Story

The inside of your penis is filled with spongy tissue. This tissue has millions of tiny spaces. Most of the time, these spaces are empty. The penis is soft. When you have an erection, blood flows into this tissue. The tiny spaces fill up with blood. This makes the spongy tissue swell. It becomes stiff and hard. The penis gets bigger and becomes erect.

An erection can happen slowly. Or it can happen in a matter of seconds. An erection can last for some time. Or it can go away quickly. It all depends on the situation. But, sooner or later, erections always go away.

How does your penis get soft again? Well, it's pretty much the opposite of getting hard. Blood flows back out of your penis. The tiny spaces in the spongy tissue empty out. Then your penis is soft again.

Erections and Puberty

66 Did I notice having them more often once puberty started? Are you kidding? I was having them all the time. 99

66 Well, I was getting boners ever since I was a kid. In fourth grade I started getting more. But it wasn't like all the time. 99

66 I remember walking around nonstop with a hard-on. 99

At times, just thinking about sex is enough to cause an erection. But erections aren't always sexual.

An erection can happen slowly. Or it can happen in a matter of seconds.

● ● ● ● ● ●

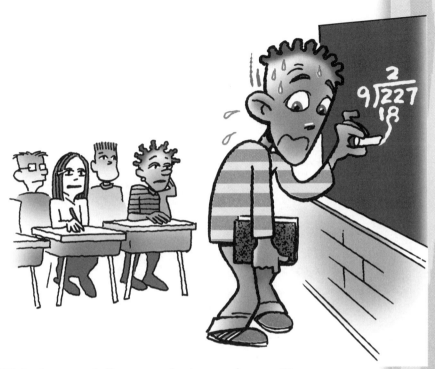

This is especially true during puberty. You may have an erection when you aren't doing or thinking about anything sexual. These are called spontaneous erections.

" I was embarrassed getting them in front of the class. "

" I'd think of things like dog poop or playing baseball. I'd take my shirt and pull it outside my pants. I'd try to cover my boner up, enough so I could walk. "

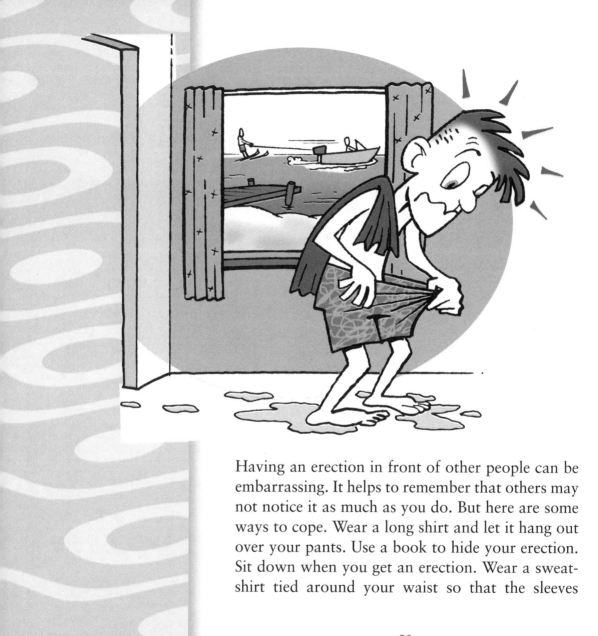

Having an erection in front of other people can be embarrassing. It helps to remember that others may not notice it as much as you do. But here are some ways to cope. Wear a long shirt and let it hang out over your pants. Use a book to hide your erection. Sit down when you get an erection. Wear a sweat-shirt tied around your waist so that the sleeves cover your front. Try to think about something else until it goes away.

The Long and Short of It

For males, penis size is a BIG issue. If you've worried about the size of yours, you're not alone! Many boys write to me about the size of their penis. In fact, I get more questions about this than anything else.

66 I always thought my penis was too small. I still do. 99

66 I look around the locker room. I think everybody has a penis bigger than mine. 99

You may think your penis is small. But, don't forget, you're still growing. Remember what you learned in Chapter 2. The penis doesn't really start to grow until Stage 3. And it doesn't reach full size until Stage 5. You've probably got a lot of growing to do.

Also, your penis can vary in size. A cold penis tends to be shorter. You may have noticed that going swimming shrinks the size of your penis.

Size differences tend to disappear when an erec-

Your penis doesn't reach full size until Stage 5. (See page 29.)
• • • • • • •

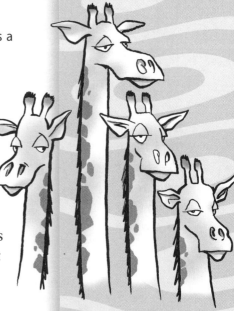

tion happens. A penis that is on the small side when soft often grows more during an erection. Penises that are long when soft tend to grow less. Maybe your soft penis *is* on the small side. But it may be normal size when you have an erection.

What about the size of the erect penis? That's a good question. Chances are, you want to know the answer.

You might think there are lots of good studies of penis size. There aren't. The best we can say is what's true for most (7 out of 10) adult men. They have erect penises between 5¼ and 6¾ inches.

Does the size of your penis really matter? The answer is no. Do people judge you on the size of your nose, or your big toe? They aren't going to judge you on the size of your penis, either. And if they do, what kind of jerks does that make them?

Do people judge you on the size of your nose, or big toe?

Do I Measure Up?

"Of course I measured mine. I wanted to be bigger. I wanted to be huge."

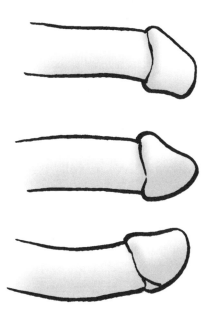

Penises come in lots of different shapes, some of which are pictured here.

• • • • • • • • •

The length of the erect penis is measured along the top. It's the distance from the point where it joins the body to its tip. Most men have measured theirs at least once in their lives. It's easy enough to do. All you need is a ruler and an erection. Lay the ruler along the top of your penis. Make your penis as straight as you can. It should be as flat as possible against the ruler. Press one end of the ruler into the pubic area at the base of your penis. Now measure the distance to the tip of the penis.

Angles and Curves

When you have an erection, your penis sticks out from your body. Some men have erections that stick up. Others have erections that stick straight out. Still other men have erections that dip down. The angle of the fully erect penis is different for different men. These differences are all perfectly normal. Of course, if you're only partly erect, it won't be the same angle as when you're fully erect.

Most erections are also straight when looked at from the side. Again, there are also many that curve. If there is a curve, it is usually up toward the body. Less often it curves down, away from the body and toward the floor.

When looked at from above, many erections are straight. But many curve a bit to the left or right. Curves are perfectly normal and quite common.

Questions & Answers

. . . .

Q **When I get an erection it hurts. The pain seems to be down near the bottom of the glans. What should I do?**

A If you have a pain when you get an erection, you should see a doctor. In fact, see a doctor if you have any pain in your penis that lasts for more than a day or so. Don't worry about being embarrassed. A doctor is trained to take care of all of your body, even that part.

Q **Is there any way to make my penis longer? My uncle told me to tie a weight on it to make it longer. Will this work?**

A No, there is no way to make your penis longer. Tying a weight to it could stretch your tissues and do serious damage. And it won't make your erect penis any longer.

Q I have an erection when I wake up in the morning. Is this normal?

A This is completely normal. In fact, erections come and go during the night while you are asleep.

Q Is it true that men with big feet have a big penis?

A No, having big feet does not mean you have a big penis. The same is true for noses, thumbs, big toes, or any other body parts.

Q My penis is long but it's skinny. Is that normal?

A Yes, that's perfectly normal. Here's the basic rule when it comes to penises: anything goes. Some penises are long. Some are short. Some are fat. Some are skinny. They are all normal.

CHAPTER 8

The Inside Story
Making Sperm and Ejaculating

• • • • • • • • • • • • • • • •

You change in many ways as you grow up. You get taller. You get heavier. Your sex organs get larger. You grow pubic and facial hair. You know when these changes are happening. You can see them with your own eyes.

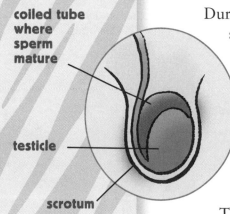

coiled tube
where
sperm
mature

testicle

scrotum

During puberty, there are also changes you can't see. They happen to the sex organs inside your body. You won't be able to see them for yourself. Even so, you will know they are happening. There will be outer signs of these inner changes.

The Testicles

During puberty the testicles grow. In Chapter 2, we talked about the testicles. They are the two egg-shaped organs inside your scrotum. You can feel them in there.

During puberty the testicles begin to make **testosterone**. Testosterone is the male sex hormone. It is just one of many hormones made in your body. Hormones are made in one part of the body. They carry messages to other parts of the body. They tell different parts of your body to grow. They also control the way your body works.

Testosterone causes the growth of the penis. It causes your muscles to grow and increases their strength. It also causes many of the other changes that you see during puberty.

Testosterone
(tes-TOS-tuh-roan)
is the male sex hormone that is made in the testicles.

Sperm

During puberty the testicles also begin making **sperm**. Sperm are the male reproductive cells. They are called reproductive cells because they allow us to reproduce. To reproduce means to make a baby. A baby starts to grow when a male reproductive cell joins with a reproductive cell from a female. Of course, even though you begin making sperm, you're not ready to be a dad. But your body is getting ready for that time in your life when you may decide to start a family.

The sperm you make are very tiny. You would need a microscope to see one. They are made inside tiny tubes in your testicles.

Each testicle is divided into hundreds of little sections. Inside each section are tiny, threadlike coiled tubes. Unwound and placed end to end, they'd reach the length of several football fields! Sperm are made inside these tiny tubes.

The sperm then move out of the testicles. They move into a larger coiled tube. There is one of these tubes on top of and behind each testicle. This is

Sperm (SPURM) is the name for the male cell that helps make a baby.

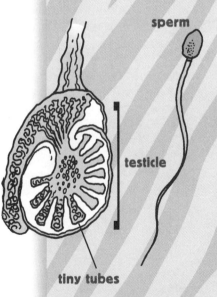

sperm

testicle

tiny tubes

where sperm are stored as they mature. You may be able to feel this tube.

During puberty, your testicles begin making sperm for the first time. They go on making sperm for the rest of your life. They make millions and millions of sperm every day. In fact, they can make as many as three million in just one hour!

Ejaculation

During puberty a boy **ejaculates** for the first time. A slang term for ejaculation is "coming." During ejaculation a mix of sperm and body fluids come out of the opening in the tip of the penis.

Here's how ejaculation works. We talked about how sperm are made in the testicles. Then they are stored in a coiled tube attached to each testicle.

A male **ejaculates** (ih-JACK-you-lates) when sperm and body fluids come out of the tip of his penis.

When a male is going to ejaculate, his penis is erect. Muscles in his sex organs go to work. These muscles pump sperm up inside of the body.

You can see how this works in the picture. There is a tube attached to each testicle. Just before ejaculation, muscles in the sex organs pump sperm from the testicles through these tubes up into the body. There the sperm in these tubes mixes with body fluids. This mixture is called **semen**. The semen is pumped

Semen
(SEE-mun) is a white fluid that contains sperm and body fluids.

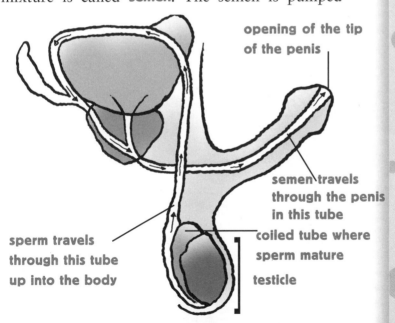

opening of the tip of the penis

semen travels through the penis in this tube

coiled tube where sperm mature

testicle

sperm travels through this tube up into the body

into yet another tube that runs the length of the penis. (Urine, or pee, also travels through this tube when it leaves the body. But urine and sperm never travel through this tube at the same time.)

During ejaculation, powerful muscle contractions pump the semen through this tube. It spurts out the opening in the tip of the penis. The semen is a creamy, white fluid. All together only about a teaspoon of semen comes out. That's not much. But it can contain 300 million to 500 million sperm!

When a man ejaculates it almost always feels good.

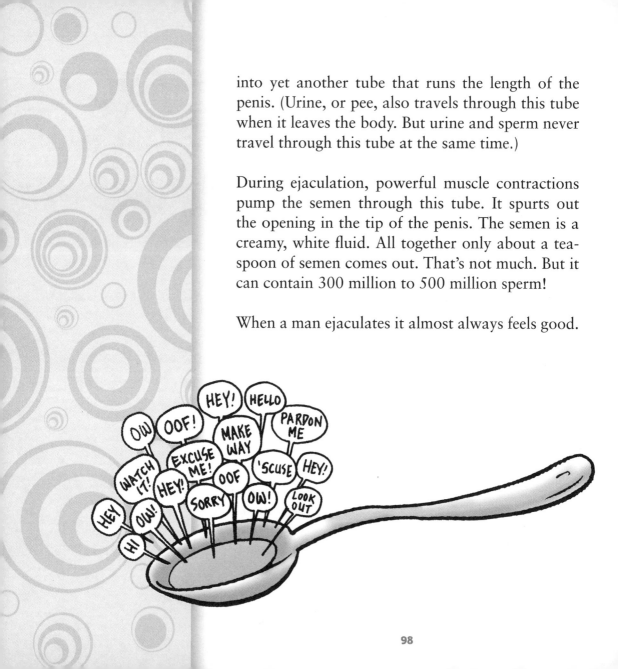

He usually has strong pleasurable feelings. This is called an orgasm. It is strongest in the sex organs. And it may spread through the body. It's hard to describe exactly how an orgasm feels. But almost everybody agrees that orgasms feel *very* good.

After ejaculation the penis gets soft again. This may happen quickly. Or it may happen slowly.

When Will I First Ejaculate?

Some boys first ejaculate early in puberty. Other boys don't start to ejaculate until later. It may be as late as Stage 5 of sex organ growth. Most boys start when they are between the ages of eleven and fifteen and a half.

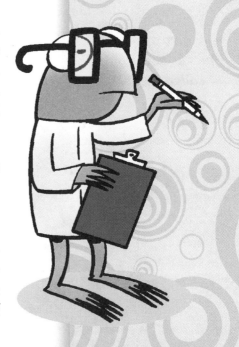

Some boys have their first ejaculation when they're asleep. When a boy ejaculates while he's asleep, it's called a wet dream.

66 Yeah, I had wet dreams. Not often, though. 99

66 I had wet dreams all the time. One time I woke up. I had such a bad wet dream, like the whole sheet was wet. It was all over the place. It was like I peed. But I knew it wasn't pee. 99

Semen can contain 300 million to 500 million sperm.

• • • •

99

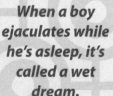

When a boy ejaculates while he's asleep, it's called a wet dream.

● ● ● ● ●

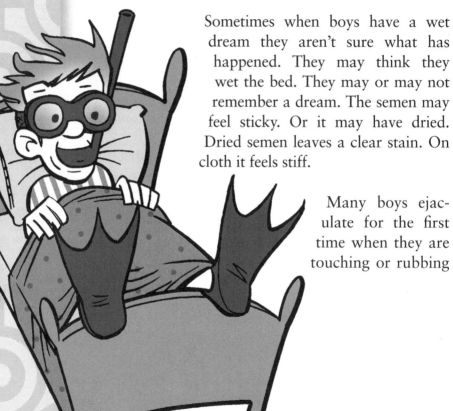

“ I don't remember having a wet dream. ”

“ I got my first wet dream. I didn't want my mom to know. I was afraid she'd see the stain on my underwear. ”

Sometimes when boys have a wet dream they aren't sure what has happened. They may think they wet the bed. They may or may not remember a dream. The semen may feel sticky. Or it may have dried. Dried semen leaves a clear stain. On cloth it feels stiff.

Many boys ejaculate for the first time when they are touching or rubbing

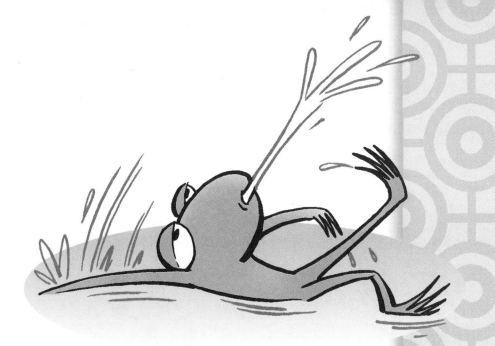

their penis. Your penis and glans are very sensitive areas. Touching yourself here usually causes an erection. And it feels good. Touching and rubbing your penis because it feels good is called masturbation. If you masturbate long enough, you will probably ejaculate. Slang terms for masturbation are "jacking off" and "playing with yourself." There are many more.

66 I used to rub it in fourth grade. I ejaculated. I kind of had a half orgasm. 99

66 No, I didn't feel embarrassed about masturbating. 99

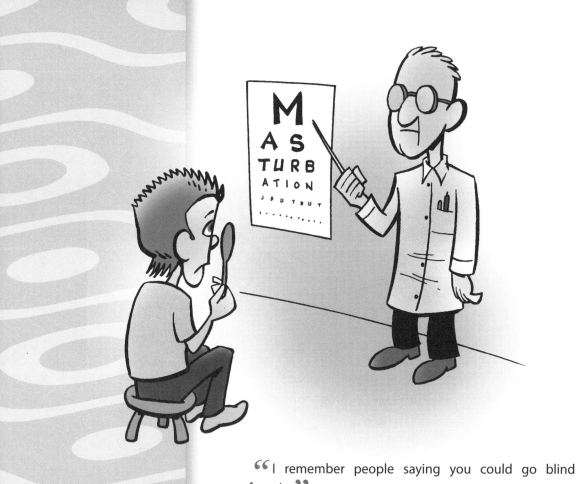

"I remember people saying you could go blind from it."

You may have heard wild stories about going blind or other terrible things that could happen if you masturbate. But masturbation won't cause any physical harm. Most boys do it at one time or another. Some boys start when they're young and continue all their lives. Others start when they are older. Some boys masturbate very often. Other boys never, or hardly ever, do. It's OK if you do and it's OK if you don't. Some people don't masturbate because of their religious or moral beliefs. And that's OK, too.

Many boys are proud when they first ejaculate. They might brag about it to their friends. You should be proud when you come for the first time. It's an important sign that you're becoming a man. You might even tell your mom or dad. You might think it would be embarrassing. Maybe if you use the word "ejaculate," it will be easier.

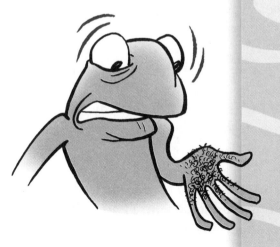

Questions & Answers

Q I was playing soccer. I got hit in my balls. That *really* hurts. So why are your testicles hanging out like that? It's too easy to have an accident.

A It's a good question, and there's a good answer. As you know, sperm are made in the testicles. To make sperm, your testicles must be at just the right temperature. This temperature is a little lower than the temperature inside your body. Inside your body, it's too warm to make sperm. So your testicles hang down in the scrotum, where it's cooler. Air flows around the scrotum, helping to keep the testicles cool.

The scrotum does its best to keep the testicles at the right temperature. If you're cold, the scrotum tightens up. This brings your testicles closer to your body. This makes them warmer. If you're hot, the scrotum hangs lower. Your testicles are further from your body. This cools them.

Q I just started to come, you know, ejaculate. I know it's supposed to be white and creamy. But my cum is clear and a little orange. How come?

A That's perfectly normal. When a boy starts to ejaculate, there aren't so many sperm in his semen. The semen is often clear and slightly yellow or orange. As you grow older you will make more sperm. Then your semen will be creamy and whiter.

Q I'm having a lot of wet dreams. How can I stop having wet dreams?

A You can't stop yourself from having wet dreams. They're just something that happens. They are completely natural and normal.

Q I've just learned about ejaculation. Semen and pee leaving the body from the same opening—oh, yuck. Is that for real?

A Yes, semen and urine do leave the body from the same opening. But it isn't yucky. They never get mixed together. They never leave the body at the same time. And that's important. Urine would kill the sperm.

Q This is kind of weird. I lost a testicle from a bike accident. Will I still be able to be a father?

A Yes. You still have one testicle. That testicle will produce plenty of sperm. Having only one testicle won't keep you from being a father.

Q I masturbate sometimes. But it doesn't "shoot" out. It just kind of dribbles out the end of my penis. Is this OK?

A Don't worry. Your ejaculations are normal. In some males, the semen never "shoots" out.

Q Sometimes I see a drop of clear fluid come out of my penis. This happens when I have an erection and before I ejaculate. What is this fluid?

A This is normal. It's called pre-ejaculatory fluid. There may be a few sperm in this fluid.

Q Sometimes my semen has some chunky or stringy pieces in it. Is this normal?

A Just after ejaculation, semen is whitish and creamy. After a few minutes, semen can change. It may then look like it has chunks or strings in it.

Q I heard that if you ejaculate too often, you can run out of sperm. Is this true?

A No, you won't run out. Every day you make millions and millions of sperm. There's just no way you can run out.

Q If you don't masturbate or have wet dreams, what happens to all those sperm?

A There's no problem. They are absorbed by the body.

CHAPTER 9

Stepping Out into the World

Becoming Your Own Self

• • • • • • • • • • • • • • • • •

As we've seen, puberty is a time of change.
Your body changes. Your feelings change.
But the changes all fit together. And you
grow from a child to a man.

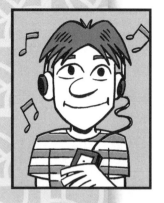
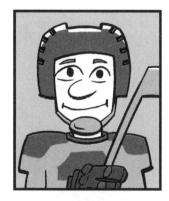
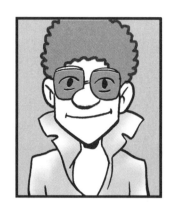

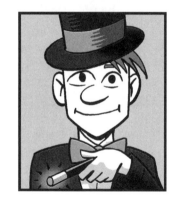
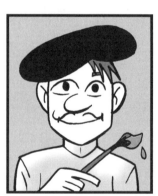

During puberty, you are becoming your own self. You get treated with more respect. You treat others with respect. You have more responsibility. You learn you have a right to your own feelings and thoughts. Your interests may change. It's all part of becoming your own self.

Puberty Is a Time of Opportunities

You will be doing new and exciting things. You will probably start going to a new school. This can be an opportunity to meet new friends. You may start new hobbies. You may get involved in sports. You may read more. You may start keeping a journal. You may have new likes and dislikes. You may like new kinds of music. You may want to choose your own clothes. You may develop your own style. You may start thinking about your future. You may have ideas about what you want to be when you grow up. You may change those ideas quite often. That's OK.

At times, you'll be pumped by all your new opportunities. At times, you may feel overwhelmed. You may think, "I don't know what I want to do." At times, you may wish for the good old days, when you were "just a kid." You may feel one way one time, and another way at another time. Feelings are like that. Knowing this is also part of growing up.

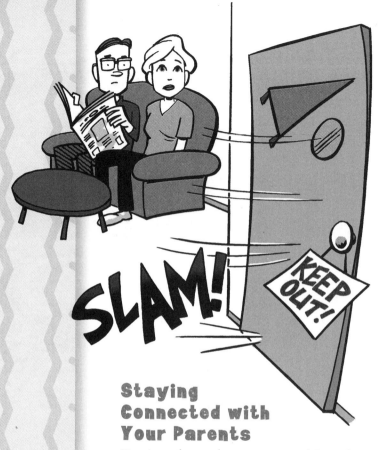

Staying Connected with Your Parents

During the puberty years, things between you and your parents change quite a bit. Before puberty, you're just a kid. Your parents take care of you. They buy your food and clothes. They keep a roof over your head. They make most of the big decisions about your life. It would be tough to survive without them. By the end of puberty, things are quite different. You're almost an adult. You may be away at school or even out on your own. You may be earning your own money. You're making more decisions for yourself. You're well on your way to being an adult. You go from being completely dependent on your parents to being almost independent. This is a big change. With this big a change, there are bound to be some problems along the way.

Puberty can be a difficult time in the way you relate to your parents. "How late can I stay out?" "Do my parents dislike my new friend?" "Do my parents respect my ideas?" "Why do I still have to go to bed early?" All of these things may come up at any time when you're growing up. But they may become bigger issues during puberty. And they may become harder to deal with.

❝They just don't understand me. ❞

You may think your parents are just "out of it." Or you may think they're too strict. At times, you may think they need to cut you some slack. But remember, your parents need to adjust to the changes, too. You may need to cut them some slack at times. Puberty is a time when you and your parents need to stay connected. So talk to them. Let them know what you are thinking and feeling. And try to listen to what they have to say.

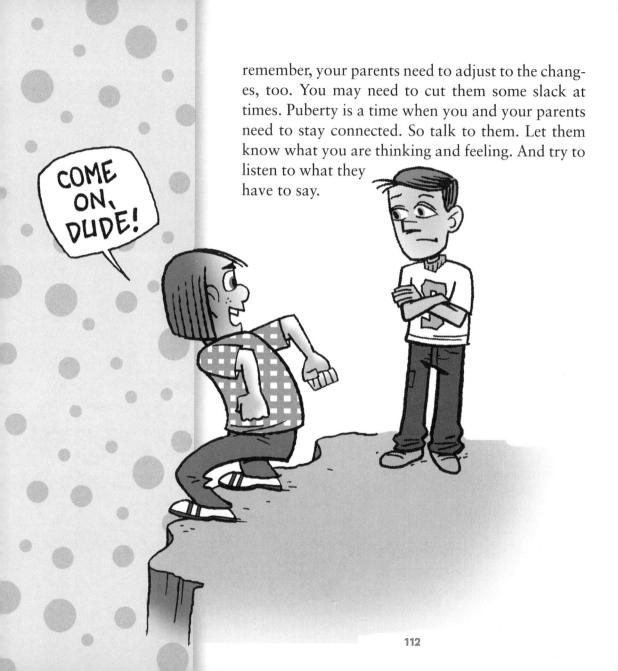

Friends

You will find new ways to relate to your friends. Having close relationships is also a part of growing up. Some boys will get crushes or romantic feelings. Others won't until later. It happens at different times for different boys.

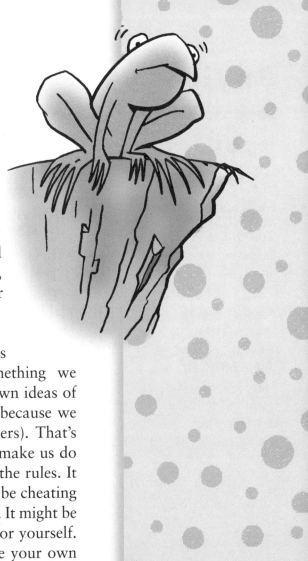

You may start hanging out with different kids. Or you may stick with all your old friends. You might want to spend lots of time with your friends. At times, you may totally need to be with your friends.

Friends can be great. But sometimes friends can talk us into doing something we shouldn't do. We may go against our own ideas of what's right and wrong. We do it just because we want to go along with our friends (peers). That's called peer pressure. Peer pressure can make us do something that's illegal, or that breaks the rules. It might be stealing from a store. It might be cheating or lying. It might be smoking a cigarette. It might be taking alcohol or drugs. Try to decide for yourself. Stand up to peer pressure. Try to make your own decisions. Don't just go along with the crowd. Don't

Saying NO to peer pressure

· · · · · · · · · · ·

Say, "No, thanks." Sometimes that's all it takes.

Keep saying no. Don't get into a debate. You don't have to defend yourself or make excuses. Just keep saying, "No, I don't want to."

(see next column ➜)

let people talk you into doing things you don't really want to do. Of course, standing up to peer pressure isn't always easy. But it is a part of becoming your own self.

Bullying and Harassment at School

You know what bullying is. It's when a kid or group of kids hurts or scares other kids. Bullies like to pick on kids who will have a hard time defending themselves. Bullying may be physical. It may involve hitting or shoving. Or it may be something that doesn't hurt physically, but hurts in other ways. It may be making mean comments or jokes. It may happen over and over.

Sexual harassment is like bullying. "Harass" means to bother. Sexual harassment means to bother in a sexual way. It can mean:

➤ Sexual comments about a person's body
➤ Sexual teasing and name calling
➤ "Pantsing" someone (pulling down their pants)
➤ Snapping towels on someone in a mean way

Everyone has the right to feel safe and happy at school. You have the right to learn, study, and join in school activities. And you have the right to do these things in a comfortable setting. Bullying gets in the way of this right. It can make it hard to pay attention in class. Or play on a sports team. Or just walk through the halls.

Too often we are told to "just ignore it" when other kids bully us. Maybe this advice works in some cases. But most of the time, "just ignoring it" doesn't work. Someone has to face up to the bully. Here are some things you can do if you are bullied, or if you see *someone else* being bullied:

• Don't be afraid to talk to an adult. This could be your mom or dad or a teacher. Be sure to tell them exactly what happened. Also tell them what would make you feel safer.

• Talk to your principal and find out how bullying is handled at your school. Ask for the principal's help. Sexual harassment is illegal. Schools have to take action to stop it.

• Don't let a bully make you feel like you are not a good person. You are. You are worthy of respect from everyone. Don't be bullied. Do what it takes to stop being bullied! And by the way, never bully or harass others.

Look the other person in the eye.
When you say no, look straight into the other person's eyes.

Use the person's name.
Say, "No, John, I don't want to do that."

If all else fails, get out of the situation.
Say, "You go ahead, I'm out of here."

You'll be surprised how effective these simple tips can be.

Abuse from Adults

Your body belongs to you. No one is allowed to abuse you physically. And no grown-up is allowed to touch you in a sexual way. It doesn't matter if that person is a parent, a relative, a friend, a minister, a rabbi, a priest, or a stranger. No one should touch you in a way that doesn't feel right to you.

If someone has touched you in this way, don't keep it a secret. No matter what happened, you haven't done anything wrong. You're the kid. No matter what anyone might say, it's not your fault. No matter what anyone might say, you don't have to protect the person who did this to you. Talk to an adult you trust. Tell the whole story. Let that person help you.

Abuse Hotline

There is a hotline set up to help young people deal with abuse. (The abuse can be sexual, physical, or emotional.) This hotline lets you talk to a trained person. You don't have to give the person your name, and it doesn't cost any money. It's called the Childhelp® National Child Abuse Hotline. The number is 1-800-422-4453 (1-800-4-A-CHILD).

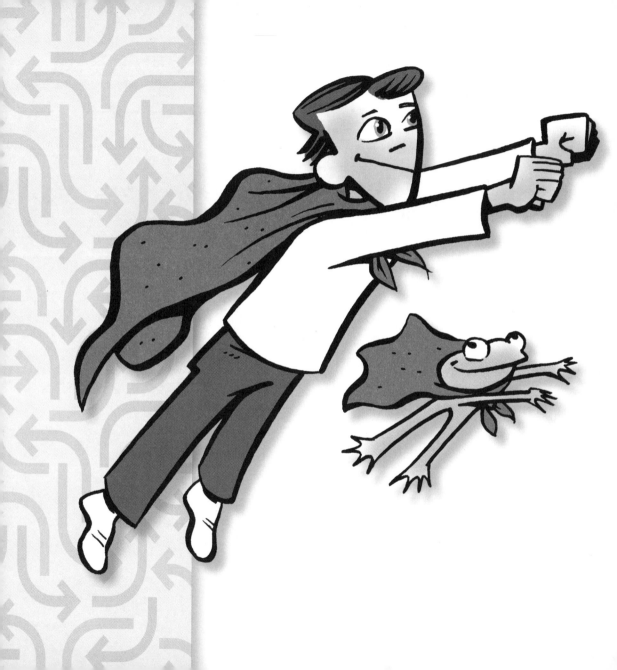

A Few Final Words

Puberty brings a lot of changes. Sometimes you will feel really good about all the changes. Sometimes you may feel pretty down. The new hormones your body is making can affect your feelings. You may have mood swings. All this is normal. But if you're feeling down, it's important to find someone to talk to. You're growing up, but you don't have to do it alone.

I hope this book has helped you. Helped you to know how your body changes. Helped you to explore your own feelings. Helped you to cope with the difficulties of growing up.

But no book is perfect. You may want to know more. You may still have questions you want answered.

So talk to people about puberty. Ask questions. Ask your parents and teachers. Ask your grandfather and other relatives. Don't be shy. Go to the library and look for other books on puberty. Find out as much as you can about this very special time in your life. **Enjoy growing up!**

INDEX

Readers Love Lynda Madaras

"I've read your book *The "What's Happening to My Body?" Book for Boys* twice already. I always found it hard talking to somebody about this subject. Your book really helped me understand and clear things up a little." —Bryan, age 14

"Your book is just fantastic, absolutely excellent...I can't believe you, a mom, knew this stuff." —Pat, age 12

"I am ten years old and read your book a little each day, and I love it. I think this is a great book and it will help a lot of people." —Jennifer, age 10

"I wanted you to know I loved your book *My Body, My Self*. It made me feel special." —Marika, age 11

"My daughter and I have spent many hours going through *The "What's Happening to My Body?" Book for Girls* and discussing many topics....Thank you for writing a wonderful book." —Leigh, mother of a 9-year-old

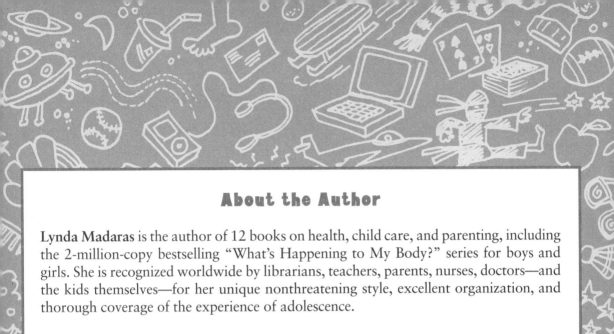

About the Author

Lynda Madaras is the author of 12 books on health, child care, and parenting, including the 2-million-copy bestselling "What's Happening to My Body?" series for boys and girls. She is recognized worldwide by librarians, teachers, parents, nurses, doctors—and the kids themselves—for her unique nonthreatening style, excellent organization, and thorough coverage of the experience of adolescence.

For more than 25 years a sex and health education teacher for girls and boys in California, she conducts workshops for teachers, parents, and librarians, and has appeared on *Oprah,* CNN, PBS, and *The Today Show.*

She wrote the first book in the "What's Happening to My Body?" series with the help of her daughter, Area, then just 11 years old and approaching puberty, and they continued to collaborate on books in the series for the next 20 years. Now a communications consultant, Area is the mother of two young girls.

The "What's Happening to My Body?" Series

THE "WHAT'S HAPPENING TO MY BODY?" BOOK FOR GIRLS

Lynda Madaras with Area Madaras

Selected as a Best Book for Young Adults by the American Library Association

In a reassuring and down-to-earth style, this book covers the body's changing size and shape; the growth spurt; breast development; the reproductive organs; the menstrual cycle; body hair; diet and exercise; romantic and sexual feelings; and puberty in the opposite sex. It also includes information on body types, anorexia and bulimia, sexually transmitted diseases, AIDS, and birth control.

288 pages. 6⅛" x 9⅛". 50 b&w drawings, bibliography, index, resources. Ages: 10 and up

ISBN: 978-1-55704-764-9. $12.95. ($14.95 Can.) pb.
ISBN: 978-1-55704-768-7. $24.95. ($29.95 Can.) hc.

MY BODY, MY SELF FOR GIRLS

Lynda Madaras and Area Madaras

This fact-filled journal and activity book makes it fun for girls to find answers to their many questions about the physical and emotional changes that accompany puberty. With quizzes, checklists, games, and illustrations throughout, *My Body, My Self for Girls* covers a wide range of topics including body image, diet, height, weight, acne, first periods and first bras. It also features journal pages and lots of personal stories addressing girls' concerns, experiences, and feelings during this new stage of their lives.

160 pages. 6⅛" x 9⅛". Over 60 b&w drawings & photos, resources. Ages: 10 and up

ISBN: 978-1-55704-766-3. $12.95. ($14.95 Can.) pb.

THE "WHAT'S HAPPENING TO MY BODY?" BOOK FOR BOYS

Lynda Madaras with Area Madaras

Selected as a Best Book for Young Adults by the American Library Association

In sensitive straight talk, this book covers the body's changing size and shape; diet and exercise; the growth spurt; the reproductive organs; body hair; voice changes; romantic and sexual feelings; and puberty in the opposite sex. It also includes information on steroid abuse, acne treatment, sexually transmitted diseases, AIDS, and birth control.

272 pages. 6⅛" x 9⅛". 48 b&w drawings, bibliography, index, resources. Ages: 10 and up

ISBN: 978-1-55704-765-6. $12.95. ($14.95 Can.) pb.
ISBN: 978-1-55704-769-4. $24.95. ($29.95 Can.) hc.

MY BODY, MY SELF FOR BOYS

Lynda Madaras and Area Madaras

This fact-filled journal and activity book makes it fun for boys to find answers to their many questions about the physical and emotional changes that accompany puberty. With quizzes, checklists, games, and illustrations throughout, *My Body, My Self for Boys* covers a wide range of topics including body image, height, weight, hair, voice changes, and perspiration. It also features journal pages and lots of personal stories addressing boys' concerns, experiences and feelings during this new stage of their lives.

128 pages. 6⅛" x 9⅛". Over 60 b&w drawings & photos, resources. Ages: 10 and up

ISBN: 978-1-55704-767-0. $12.95. ($14.95 Can.) pb.

READY, SET, GROW!
A "What's Happening to My Body?" Book for Younger Girls
Lynda Madaras

Alternate selection, Children's Book-of-the-Month Club

In age-appropriate language, this book is written especially for 8- to 11-year-old girls and is illustrated with playful and lively two-color cartoon drawings throughout.

"Upbeat, reassuring...A friendly, accessible introduction to puberty that young girls can read alone, not just with parents." —*Booklist*

"A timely and important book." —*School Library Journal* (starred review)

**128 pages. 7" x 7". 40 color illustrations, index.
Ages: 8 and up**

ISBN: 978-1-55704-565-2. $12.00. ($14.00 Can.) pb.
ISBN: 978-1-55704-587-4. $22.00. ($26.00 Can.) hc.

ON YOUR MARK, GET SET, GROW!
A "What's Happening to My Body?" Book for Younger Boys
Lynda Madaras

The newest addition to the *"What's Happening to My Body?"* series, this book is written in age-appropriate language for 8- to 11-year-old boys and is illustrated with fun and lively two-color cartoon drawings throughout.

**128 pages. 7" x 7". 75 color illustrations, index.
Ages: 8 and up**

ISBN: 978-1-55704-781-6. $12.00. ($14.00 Can.) pb.
ISBN: 978-1-55704-780-9. $22.00. ($26.00 Can.) hc.

MY FEELINGS, MY SELF
A Growing-Up Guide for Girls
Lynda Madaras and Area Madaras

Allowing a young girl to explore her questions and feelings about herself, her parents, and her friends, this popular workbook/journal provides answers, along with stories and letters from teens and preteens expressing their feelings about what's going on in their lives.

**160 pages. 7¼" x 9". 30 drawings. Bibliography.
Ages: 10 and up**

ISBN: 978-1-55704-442-6. $12.95. ($14.95 Can.) pb.

THE "WHAT'S HAPPENING TO MY BODY?" SERIES
BY LYNDA AND AREA MADARAS

Order from your local bookstore, or write or call: Newmarket Press, 18 East 48th Street, New York, NY 10017; (212) 832-3575 or (800) 669-3903; Fax (212) 832-3629; E-mail sales@newmarketpress.com

Please send me the following books:

THE "WHAT'S HAPPENING TO MY BODY?" BOOK FOR GIRLS
_____ copies at $12.95 each (paperback)
_____ copies at $24.95 each (hardcover)

THE "WHAT'S HAPPENING TO MY BODY?" BOOK FOR BOYS
_____ copies at $12.95 each (paperback)
_____ copies at $24.95 each (hardcover)

MY BODY, MY SELF FOR GIRLS
_____ copies at $12.95 each (paperback)

MY BODY, MY SELF FOR BOYS
_____ copies at $12.95 each (paperback)

READY, SET, GROW!
A "What's Happening to My Body?" Book for Younger Girls
_____ copies at $12.00 each (paperback)
_____ copies at $22.00 each (hardcover)

ON YOUR MARK, GET SET, GROW!
A "What's Happening to My Body?" Book for Younger Boys
_____ copies at $12.00 each (paperback)
_____ copies at $22.00 each (hardcover)

MY FEELINGS, MY SELF
A Growing-Up Guide for Girls
_____ copies at $12.95 each (paperback)

For postage and handling, add $5.00 for the first book, plus $1.50 for each additional book. Please allow 4–6 weeks for delivery. Prices and availability subject to change.

I enclose a check or money order, payable to Newmarket Press, in the amount of $_____.

Name _____

Address _____

City/State/Zip_____

Special discounts are available for orders of five or more copies. For information, contact Newmarket Press, Special Sales Dept., 18 East 48th Street, New York, NY 10017; (212) 832-3575 or (800) 669-3903; Fax (212) 832-3629; E-mail sales@newmarketpress.com   www.newmarketpress.com

On Your Mark 04/2008